Macrobiotics

Ph.D. Benjamin Schmidt Dis.

There is already a period in life when one could rest with
folded hands. A high work performance is required from him
together from school {years to high|high years to} age.
Most developed countries set the retirement age for men at
sixty five years. In our country! At sixyone, the average man
only eats about a month longer. So they should work until
the end of their life. All this {requires the ability to
change|the ability that is required} your life style
according to the given conditions.
Lifestyle is largely made up of diet.
After all, {World Health Organization statistics|World that
is health statistics} are uncompromisingly convinced of
this. We occupy the place of the tail of the monitored
countries in the length of the average age.

1

That's for consideration. It seems to be too {high tax on tradition|tradition that are high tax}
Speaking of traditions, let's clarify that they are as long as we think. In ancient times, we, like all other European peoples, started with roasted grain bream, wild vegetables, meat and plain ovoel. Then came the time of {cereal porridges,|cereal porridges} which, however, have certain disadvantages when traveling. They could not be transported, sour Therefore, people resorted to baking flatbreads. At first unleavened Early Middle Ages {however already caught up with us} with bread in hand, many different kinds were made from different cereals and other substitute ingredients. Some types were nothing like today's bread. As long as the Guilds were not destroyed by mass, there was plenty of food; meat from hunting deer, fish, vegetables, cereals. Individual European countries thrived only on the popularity of one or another cereal. In Bohemia, millet ruled, in Moravia buckwheat ruled. They were supplemented by now-forgotten vegetables such as turnips, turnips, parsnips and {self- grown cabbage that is self-grown}. Root

vegetables are {eaten like later potatoes| later potatoes that is eaten as}. The age of potatoes came only after the Thirty Years' War, when the country was looted, destroyed and the nation suffered from famine. The imported potato, with its sufficient amount of starch and vitamins, saved the Guilds from {death by hunger. White flour, called Hungarian flour, appeared at the end of the last century and {made it possible to bake bread|baked that are made possible} so it was known from the castle. shaply and soft.. Root vegetables are {eaten like later potatoes|later potatoes that is eaten as}. The age of potatoes came only after the Thirty Years' War, when the country was looted, destroyed and the nation suffered from famine. The imported potato, with its sufficient amount of starch and vitamins, saved the Guilds from {death by hunger. White flour, called Hungarian flour, appeared at the end of the last century and {made it possible to bake bread|baked that are made possible} so it was known from the castle. Bflé and soft.. Root vegetables are {eaten like obd later potatoes| obd later potatoes that is eaten as}. The age of potatoes came only after the Thirty Years' War,

3

when the country was looted, destroyed and the nation suffered from famine. The imported potato, with its sufficient amount of starch and vitamins, saved the Guilds from {death by hunger. White flour, called Hungarian flour, appeared at the end of the last century and {made it possible to bake bread|baked that are made possible} so it was known from the castle. Bflé and soft.. called Hungarian, it was built at the end of the last century and {made it possible to bake bread|baked that are made it possible} so it was known from the castle. Bflé and soft.. called Hungarian, it was built at the end of the last century and {made it possible to bake bread|baked that are made it possible} so it was known from the castle. Bflé and soft..

As we can see, the Czech nation has always shown enough respect for the national cuisine. According to rumour his habits. I think it's time {again not|se that is again} a problem to think

At the beginning of this century, with the increased consumption {quin white flour,| flour that is quin white} of fatty meats, with the onset of industrial processing of food, the first warning voices of dietitians appeared. To be

precise, doctors before reason
they have been warning with food since
ancient times. However, it was mainly about
the behavior of rich people, whom the advice
concerned. In our century {the warning has
begun|the warning that is} applies to
everyone. Doctors pointed out! and the
necessary use of unbleached flour and
naturally
eating vegetables. The names of some
European die-fologh are not forgotten to this
day. They also celebrated great {successes
like|like that is success} 16-year-olds, but the
progression of problematic foods
failed to stop. Even after the Second World War,
doctors continued to create chisel systems that
preyed on many sick people. At that time, an
interesting dietary system called macrobiotics
penetrated Europe and the USA".
The exporting country this time was Japan. At
first, macro-
was presented as a therapeutic diet, and only
later were other elements of oriental {ált
adravovédy,|adravovédy that is ált} assigned
to the art of cooking and eating, such as the art
of breathing, massages and gymnastics. he was
Japanese, known in Western countries as

George Oshawa. In the 1960s, he published and lectured in Europe on ikebana, acupuncture, Japanese martial arts. Besides. he also published the book Zen-macrobiotics, in which he describes ways to preserve or restore a person's health by preparing food based on the principles of Far Eastern philosophy. The name-robiotics was chosen very thoughtfully, because in the language it means "big life", and this is a dream that {certainly goes as far|so that is certainly reaches} as long as the cultural history of mankind. Macro-meal in Oshaw's concept was a strict diet. Depending on the treacherous state, the patient could tighten his diet from dullness, which was the most benevolent, up to the 7th stage, when the ship's diet consisted of {exclusively whole-grain rice| rice that is exclusively whole-grain}.

According to {literary data|data that is literary}, this man died at the age of 72 from lung cancer, when he spent the last years of his life in the Lombardy in the collective of the world-famous humanist Dr. Albert Schweitzer. Oshawa, however, {he left a dream-|a dream that is left behind} when he spent the last years of his life in the Lombard in the collective of the world-famous humanist Dr. Albert Schweitzer. Oshawa, however, {he left a dream-|a dream that is left behind} when he spent the last years of his life in the Lombard nonice in the collective of the world-famous humanist Dr. Albert Schweitzer. Oshawa, however, {he left a dream-|a dream that is left behind}

Bucks. We will be most interested in the personality of Michio Kushi, who settled on the east coast of the USA and founded the Foundation West-Ost, which is commercially very Hi Near Boston in the USA, he runs a macrobiotic trum-Kushi Institute, where people gather from all over to study macrobiotics. Kushi's Japanese wife Avelina runs Aveline's Makrobiotic Natural Food Store. Viasta {publishing house publishes dozens|publishes that is publishing house} of subtitled titles.

Robotics. In a number of US cities, restaurants and stores focused on macrobiotic food are being created. However, it cannot be concluded that macrobiotics have taken over the United States and America

7

You see, it is actually impossible to write a good macrobiotic cookbook. You can only raise a good macrobio {cook or cookbook|or a cookbook that is a cook}. The magic is in the person and in
Macrobiotic plate
Macrobiotic cookbooks never presuppose recipes for {a whole menu|a menu that is whole}. He eats his macrobiotics during the day, at most the day before. According to
{currently, the cook chooses, for example, cereals|who the cook chooses, for example, cereals that is current}. The season offers him
{different types of vegetables|different types of vegetables that is not}. Method preparation is given by time or health status. Macrobiotics is therefore a very creative way of eating. It forces a person to rethink his condition and lifestyle, to put them together with the menu. It has its own advantage. A person's health lies in his hands. He loses anxiety and fear of the unknown, which lies beyond his reach.
The macrobiotic plate has a standard form and some {rich variant|variant that is rich}. In

the framework of this publication {we will be concerned in, that is} the more frequent composition of the daily diet. When we talk about biotic strall, we have an idea of the composition of the diet day by day

Half of the daily {food intake to make up whole grain lunch|make up whole grain lunch that is food intake}. They are mostly prepared in the form of unprocessed grains. A smaller percentage {can be processed|be that is } into raugh things like flakes or whole wheat flour. A third of the plate is made up of vegetables. Macrobiotical person chews as healthy only those vegetables that come from the zone in which the person currently lives. Vegetables very rich assortment of taste, color and effects. Predominantly represented both thermally processed raw greens, but also vegetables {treated with lactic acid|lactic acid that is treated}.

The third {part of the macrobiotic plate| macrobiotic that is part} are legumes, they are a source of valuable protein. Their share is 10%. In a year, 5 kg of macrobiotics are added to the diet when there is no meat on the plate.

In small quantities, they supplement talif seeds, including They are a source of high-

9

quality oil. Of course, fat is also often necessary. We will talk about that later. Well, the seeds are available, we have to use more fat to pay for the whole day. In the opposite case, we add seed of castor bean, lau, pumpkin or sesame. Seeds also change the taste of food, which is why they often replace roots.

14

is less important for {macrobiotics|less that is macrobiotics} than vegetables. mainly during the ripening period. That is, from early summer Outside of this period {the macrobiotic prefers| the macrobiotic that is gives} the subject, baked or stewed before fresh or

but an important supplement are wild vegetables, waj {mineral content|mineral that is content} and other compo- region in our environment seaweed, used

nations. The most widespread are nettle, plantain leaves, husf sedge, daisy, dandelion roots. Fantasies may not be true. Furthermore, edible plants! Also the spices of {our grandmothers for|grandmothers that is our} macrobiotic renaissance. Lovage, calamint, sage, balka, marjoram, muskwort, wild marjoram, mate - these are interesting and healthy macrobiotic supplements -

to the fact that the birthplace of macrobiotics is Japan, Asian cat is quite often popular in cooking. It is considered a medicine in Asian countries. We use an adaptogen, i.e. a substance that improves the juice from the fresh root has the best effects. However, it is not yet available on our market.

hey

we can't forget the meat. Someone is a vegetarian. Surprisingly, I know hundreds of people who are so presto {enjoy excellent health|excellent health that is enjoyable} Others do it without Dr. In that case, macrobiotics recommend moderation. In itself, however, macrobiotics is not a way of eating. It is a teaching about the influence of diet on the balance of human life. macrobiota-eats meat two to three times a week. Preference. ryld and meat of other aquatic animals. There are other

farthest. Also, the meat of birds and poultry is considered by rebiotics to be less harmful than the meat of mammals. In the diet it means to cut out pork, Carnivorous animals do not eat at all. If it is in a colder environment or we are doing feast work, we

add more meat. If we have to situselch
when we have to eat meat, we will give
priority an animal's hide before a long-lived
animal.
Bijlci game is better than an animal fattened in
the
cotton wool with stronger spices and
vegetables. Served with vegetable salads,
mustard seeds, ill and the like, to avoid
negative effects- {they arise during
digestion| they arise during digestion that is
ré}.

gie is distributed in the organism according to
the precise schemes of individual organs
individual that and other schemes} and thus
revives the organism. This is where another
malfunction occurs. The paths for the life-
giving woman can be impassable, the organs
overloaded or even without energy. It is
possible to revive these pathways {with the
help of diet|heal that is with}, exercise,
psychological action, breath, but also with
drugs, massages, the intervention of a metal
needle, i.e. a puncture, or a knife, i.e.
surgically..

Suddenly, a medic of the oriental
understanding of man opens before us.
The

disease is caused by changes in the environment in which we live, by the influence of negative psychological stimuli, but also by our laziness in breathing and diet. S is to keep the organism in good harmony and only tune it with daily interventions, for example with herbs or a change of diet with physical relaxation, rather than correcting severe disorders that mimic disease. If the organism does not have enough defenses, the disease cannot be prevented, or the disease becomes chronic.

Practical macrobiotics

Many words lose their meaning without practice. Let's show how our own macrobiotic diet is created.

The aforementioned dietitians with {noticed certain connections|certain that is noticed} the increasing incidence of degenerative mental and other diseases and the change in the assortment and processing of positive foods.

He took advantage of: a certain depression of humanity due to feelings of alienation from nature, which is manifested today, for example, by someone's interest in ecology, and offered America and Europe a sustainable system based on the above assumptions. symptoms of aging, such as joint wear and tear, multiple sclerosis, spinal mobility disorders, kidney and ear stones and many other diseases, but also a feeling of wear and tear, gout, depression, non- kiids, and anxiety. This means a lot for {mankind|many that is mankind}. Propagató {but the blots were talking|but that is blots} also about something, which sounds unbelievable to our European ears. About the fact that macrobiotics will improve the quality of life, because a person has become gentler, more understanding, more balanced. This is essential tal nutrition and macrobiotics. Small nutrition is completely sufficient to reduce the risk of heart disease or the risk of developing tumors.

Macrobiotics is sou ent philosophy of life, gives it a certain content, proto- grasses nevid! joules, minerals, fats or vi als through food shapes a person's view and through food he thinks about his perfect - and this is really possible, I'll leave it up to everyone's - life. {wa read out to the world,|Wa read out to the world} that he violated the laws of natural balance - people consume a significant amount of artificially produced dogs, drugs and chemicals, manure artificial fertilizers, plants are poisoned by insecticides and herbicides, feed hormones and antibiotics. A large part of the diet consists of foods such as {refined sugar,|sugar that is refined} preparations. The most

they sinned by disturbing the balance of the cereal Te formed {the basis of human diet for thousands of years|human diet for thousands of years that is the basis}. In na- et, however, people threw away the husk of the grain and consumed only the non-food fire. Oshawa also disagreed with that

have fruits and vegetables grown in a different temperature than 2111. {This then causes an imbalance, the disintegration of the organism and thus the emergence of mental or physical carries as well as the deterioration of interpersonal relationships and the relationship to pre- Hacrobiotics should therefore avoid eating drugs and ky of prepared substances, refined sugar, tropical crops and white flour| And thus also the emergence of mental or physical carries also the deterioration of

interpersonal relationships and the relationship to pro- Hacrobiotics should therefore avoid eating drugs and ky of prepared substances, refined sugar, tropical crops and white flour then causes an imbalance, dis- t of the organism}. He should be looking for {food that is food|food that are food}
natural conditions, presto chemical. Even in such foods the balance was not disturbed - Ja Jang. We can demonstrate such a balance - for example, on a cereal grain. That is {consists in principle|in principle that is consists}.
t. The inner part of the grain, represented by starch and starch, i.e. gluten, is yin. Around it
is a shell containing minerals, indigestible fiber, etc.
he is yang. The reviving element is the key. Let's inflate the package and the key. We will destroy its viable-balanced grain and make it almost exclusively a source of Milkovyna.
We will create a diet from it that has dcinek of a different character. With long-term use-- this imbalance takes its revenge. In order for everyone to really understand philosophy, the authors of the vysingan, according to which we can choose individual ones. you are what

you eat, you are what you
eat." 10
11

When choosing an oil, macrobiotics recommends using pr la jm-yang. The smaller the seed the oil is extracted from, the more yang properties. At the top of this rating are my oil and {flexible oil|flexible that is oil}. They are very suitable for winter. In summer, we use sunflower and soybean oil. {Plant oil is suitable for a very hot day|Day plant oil is suitable for a very hot day}. Olive oil is a macrobiotic from the temperate zone, very low.

Unsuitable foods

In macrobiotics, very few foods are strictly no. Chemically prepared foods, drugs, and raw sugar are among those to which macrobiotics are known. Be careful not to make a mistake, Sweet in macrobiotics is on the contrary desirable. The source of sweetness must be refined sugar from Sugar Pepa and not cane.

Tolerated {not even grape sugar|sugar that is not even} or mec simple sugars have never in the history of Clove been zoomed even in a tenth of the amount that is common at the time.

In macrobiotics, sugar is referred to as a source of physical and {mental difficulties| difficulties that is mental}. It is addictive, like a drug.

Addiction to sugar can have the character of addiction.

The list of {negative properties of sugar| properties that is negative} would exceed the corner of this publication. It is considered very important that sugar creates a strongly acidic reaction in the body, which not only causes ulcers and inflammations on the lining of the intestines, but also drains {reserves of minerals| mineral substances that is reserves}.

Calcium, hot elements take part in the alkalization of acid-forming sugars, such as minerals, trace elements and vitamins. Our diet, however, is limited by these components to artificially produced vitamins and substances that the body needs to incorporate into the body, thus creating a carousel {strikingly reminiscent of the gic effect|gical that is strikingly reminiscent} of man in nature.

Sugar is found in many food products. It can be found in milk products, pastries, jams and stews or liqueurs. Excess sugar is a complex {costa in fatty|in fatty that is costa} acid. These change not only the appearance of the clos but also the function of many organs. At the same time, sugars, exactly gla| gla that is them} essential for the functioning of the nervous and muscular apparatus- sugar in the blood causes fatigue and disorders. However, the organism is ideally equipped to break down simple sugars. Their smooth transformation {supplying the nervous system with the necessary|Supplying the system that is nervous} pall that we live mainly on animal proteins and Borgenism convert these necessary glucose in a complex way. This consumes energy, then it is missing elsewhere. The balance is broken.

ka considers refined sugar to be an extreme yin In the spirit of oriental health science, it reduces resistance to diseases, affects nervous activity. encourage the emergence of {allergic diseases|diseases that are allergic}. Stej also likes artificial sweeteners.

lik rad {pro macrobiotics|macrobiotics that is pro}

the flaw used to be very subtle. She noticed an unusual detail that the Europeans generously overlooked. and on which we prepare food, we can't. The most suitable is a fire made of wood, least of all microwaves.

ob from more natural materialsà, the better. Kera much preferred over {plastic or aluminum|or aluminum that is plastic}.

they maintain their activity only for a limited time. arno has been of the same quality for years. Flour only them Vegetables for several days. The fresher the food, the more effective it is.

science has become an integrator of biological cultivation This is the cultivation of agricultural crops, vegetables and Bit chemicals, antibiotics and hor-

grasses are gaining great popularity in the world and l- ani {their higher price|higher that is theirs}, Pada statki at vi biological cultivation of cereals and vegetables here too, {the most suitable foods for a sick person,|The most suitable foods for a sick person are those that are kept close to his place of residence. It is said that a person needs the least strength to bathe.

cook in good health and with love. Negative el- Oriental traditions are passed on through diet. concentrated and above all slowly. What a

person is. {the longer he has to chew the food|
The longer he has to chew the food that is
longer}. It helps with anxiety and does not
deplete his energy.

18

13

Eggs are used only occasionally, depending on
age. Macrobiotics store one egg per week.
Preference {maj from fowl|from that is maj}
21ffcf outside and from fowl inseminated.
Liquids form a separate chapter. In general, we
drink less, but not a little. However, the fluid
intake is relatively high. Is it a paradox? We
go to his Felon when we realize that boiled
vegetables contain a considerable amount of
water in themselves. C amount of fluid
received is therefore the same for all {hy
eating|eating that is hy}. It just depends on
what form p me. We supplement the need for
free fluids with high-quality purified water,
herbal teas, and cereal coffees. The bar rem is
that we are not thirsty and that we do not
urinate more than 4- in 24 hours.
A word about other foods
Salt is an essential part of food preparation. Jo,

however, poses a danger to human health. First of all, the relationship between salt and high blood pressure is detailed. In the macro, sa, together with fire and pressure, belongs to the important yang ments. Salt {gives food yang tendency|food yang tendency that is provides}.

It brings important {mineral substances| substances that is mineral} into the ganism. Nevertheless, salt consumption is minimal in the macrobium. It is always consumed in a bound me, i.e. in one that has undergone boiling. Ready-made food {ticky is never salted|never that is ticky}, with one exception, which will be discussed later. The macrobiotic's consumption of salt is somewhat smaller than is customary in our civilization.

One of the reasons for low consumption is undoubtedly serious health problems, such as strokes and perhaps 1 stomach cancer, which are attributed to high consumption in Japan.

The macrobiotic prefers sea salt, which contains a lot of trace elements {than salt refined|refined that is than salt}. As said, macrobiotics took over from {eastern nations| nations that is eastern} macrobiotics

to solent preparations produced by
fermentation with

mountain solf. The most famous are the Tat Shoyu soy sauces. Miso soy paste, which goes by many trade names, is very popular. The specific preparation for sloths is called Gomasto. We will prepare it by roasting the hungry ko in a {dry pan|a pan that is dry}. Roasted cost seeds

14

Fine powder. We will do the same separately with the mol- Ongredience mixed in a ratio of 8:1 to 12:1 in Gomaslo becomes ready on the table and {salted j directly|j that is salted} on the plate. It also brings fat in optimal sik soll causes a feeling of tiredness, lack of appetite, etc

tra sol causes excessive thirst, sleepless mental stiffness, a feeling of heaviness in the back. without fat it is difficult to prepare daily meals.

Fats bring a number of essential nutrients to the body

a well-known source of energy and {by heating them suitable|by heating that is their} conditions for thermal processing of food- Slovakia, however, we have such a consumption of fats, which exceeds the amount necessary for health. Fats. avame primarily {in

hidden form|hidden that is in}. They are {in large|large that is in}
in meats, sausages, fatty cheeses and eggs. en consumption of fats is one of the important facto-. aclerotic manifestations in blood vessels. Fats are often associated with a disease we call heart attack - Heat treatment of fats leads to the formation of substances that provoke the development of malignant tumors. Also, cooking oil and fats are related to each other.

dantive many reasons for macrobiotics to include fats. It is only an apparent impression.

Fats

e for the smooth running of body functions, strength sy| function of strength sy that is ných}. Our nerve cells need vitamin Pat malova, which belongs to unsaturated fatty acids. We find these mainly in vegetable fats, when
{in the diet a smaller amount|In a smaller that are diet} of quality plants- and our thinking abilities can deteriorate. Heklad lecithins, which we can get from some
oil, is priceless for the organism. The best unsaturated fatty acids are the seeds of nettle,

other and {sesame seed|seed that is sesame}.
Also ote-
large amounts of oil. Therefore, in
macrobiotics. dla likes to use only a very small
amount of flax, the mentioned seeds are
added, nuts no- {ndemnice olejné|olejné that
are ndemnice}.
ka clearly prefers oils obtained by pressing -
Such oil has the disadvantage that it oxidizes
quickly. Therefore, it does not fit into the
{regular sales network|regular sales network}.
Popular for oils from vegetable sprouts.
macrobiotic regulations strictly reject
fats.
Macrobiotics has reservations about saturated
fats. Pinching occurs to some, for both
macrobiotics and reaction.
17

rican. It is only one of dozens of diets that are
fighting for popularity. I mention the name
Kushi because this under coffee man has
created a number of branches in European
countries. Pe runs bombastic courses for
thousands of interested people in
Switzerland, advertises summer camps,
founded a school whose graduates get
diplomas. Since it is a

company that lives only on its earnings, it can be concluded that it is economically viable due to the solid interest in this way of life.

Principles of macrobiotics

As already stated, macrobiotics is a response to an overexamined society. He tries {in his principles|his that is ve} to turn to a natural way of life. She gained popularity above all by publishing positive treatment results for difficult-to-read diseases, including malignant tumors. Science has not fully confirmed these findings, on the contrary, critical articles have been published in a number of journals, for example reports on the defective development of children fed strict macrobiotics. of the current inhabitants of the planet Earth This is of course not a problem, because every learning you Man has become extremely {separated from nature|from nature that is separated}. At first, that fact filled him with pride and {pride of his|his that are pride} of womanhood. Later, he felt the fear of his loneliness and then 21 after becoming an integral part of it again. Man observes nature, sees its immortality. Flowing water, you are Like soft grass or an old tree, still renewing

their lively powers. If man merges with nature, he gains something of its resistance to extinction. The ancient Chinese philosophy of Taoism taught how to do it practically. Tao means the path. Whoever walks the path of tao learns to perceive things wisely and is able to bring himself into harmony with everything that exists. In apparent chaos, he finds a way that knows the order of all being. In this {several thousand year old|year that is several thousand} Chinese f fi is to be sought for the true roots of macrobiotic soba life. With macrobiotics, we don't have to be afraid of these religious circles, Macrobiotics has nothing to do with religion. It's not about worshiping any god, prayers, ord ni, waiting for a miracle {whether spasent|spasent that is or}. We don't even have to deal with the actual background of the mak blottka at all.
Japanese people
us with their pragmatic thinking, because they were able to howl from their rie connected with a special upbringing of individuals. vim realistic and practical conclusions. Today them, as well as. ye Oriental sages, it is about the constant reproduction of life-forces, the

preservation of health, and the loss of
anxiety from separation from
Therefore, in the system of macrobiotics, they
created {practically k jed|k that is practically}
one of the possible life philosophies. on the
way {tao says,|says that is tao} that everything
around us, even everything in the distant
cosmos exists only thanks to the ever-
intertwining har- of two forces. In the apparent
chaos, we can find the order of everything only
when we understand the essence of the
constant harmony of these Chans, since the
time of the founder of Taoist teachings, Lao-
Tzu, call these forces Yin and Yang. These are
words whose
infinitely wide. They indicate principles that
are contradictory. If we were to bring them
closer to each other, then I {show graphically
with mathematical signs|show that is
graphically} signs and Ho with the words man
and woman, or any terms that stand in
opposition. However, the following sentences
are very important for {understanding the
macro|macro- that are understanding}. When
reading these fá-, we will immediately
imagine that one principle, marked with an
amen +, is

positive, good and beneficial, while the principle marked has a negative influence. This leads to dualism, which we overcome only with the greatest difficulty. {the yang concept of macrobiotics is|the yang of macrobiotics that is concept} one, indivisible.

That is why we cannot label one in macrobiotics. Poor and second to good. There is only food, according to the Yin and Yang principle, it is either harmonious with {our st,| st that is our} environment and with nature, or disharmo- In such a case, a person who invites disharmony finds himself in conflict with the environment and balance. allob, perhaps at the cost of illness or bad behavior. iontain medicine was medi-energetic in today's sense of the word. The predominance of contemporary research on orlen-| with that is né research} of the blochemic area. This is just for clarification

the difference between our and oriental thinking. Duty-- according to the ideas of Orlent {surrounded by many forces|mnoha that is surrounded}, who works unconditionally.

The main influence st preserves the cosmos. Stly of these two

also indirectly, thanks to inhaled inflammable food. If we were very perfect, we would only use the energy of the cosmos and the earth, but we get our energy through the great air and food. One person exhales 700 kg a year and digests 600 {kg of food|food that is kg}. This huge tet 14tek has a significant influence on a person. The obtained energy

Macrobiotics and {current science|the science that is current}

The development of nutrition science is very dynamic. Some that were valid a decade ago are no longer valid today. An important part of human nutrition research is to prevent even the harmful effects of an inadequate diet, it is {sice dox,|dox that is sice} that millions of people in the world die precisely because of poor nutrition. Some starving. others by overeating.
Nevertheless, it is the scientist's responsibility to prevent the spread of fanatical diets that could harm health. Indeed, research has also found that strictly {observed macrobiotics in| macrobiotics that is observed} in infants and young children leads to a slowdown in physical growth and to a slowdown in lower

development. It is a bit different when a person has been eating a certain food for many generations or when a change means too sudden a transition for him. Therefore, we do not recommend macrobs for children. However, some sets are suitable.

However, even an adult must be careful about his health. He who does not want to really devote himself to nutrition and stick to the principles of {rational nutrition|nutrition that is rational}. For the sake of his health, he will give it up. However, if he wants to achieve {in his mental|his that is in} both physical and military higher goals, then he can continue his studies. They mainly concern food, Mase ka and potatoes. There is no place for scientific solutions, p mo. When consuming! macrobiotic meals, however, it is difficult to realize some connections,

blood

Many people are able to live without meat or with a small amount of it. For others, such a life means danger, carefully monitoring their health. First of all, the hormonal cycle and the levels of iron and calcium. For that reason, we are attaching {tables of content of some foods|

content of some foods that is tables}.
The second friction surface is milk. Nutritional science recommends milk primarily for protein and calcium. Milk was never consumed in Ciò and Japan. Bohemia is {on the contrary the homeland of shepherds|the homeland of shepherds that is on the contrary}. Except that our tolerance to milk is already well {genetically conditioned|treated that is genetically}. It is therefore significantly better {than Asian|that is than} the nation, a number of Czechoslovak macrobiotics supplement it with some dairy products, such as sheep and goat hard cheeses, cottage cheese and fermented milk products Czechoslovak supplement of macrobiotics. Health and age are taken into account. It is also important to note that we do not have soy protein such as Natto soy milk, Tofu cottage cheese or cheese available. They are not macrobiotics of Arana. Only their consumption is essentially a lack of fiber and a strong jinn.
Japanese or American macrobiotics can be an inspiration, but not a dogma. Hem are

historically associated with the consumption of more protein, leavened bread and, finally,

{even with stvi|with that is even} good beer, a
healthy person does not have to completely
Rification of food according to yin-yang
principles
foodstuffs
opposites
foodstuffs
{hove selentna products,|hove selentna that is
products} celery and natively grown
and pressed
and oils and seeds isoated and mjet teas and
spring water
● nuts
● fruit from our climate zone malt
syrup Strongly yin foods
●
white flour
husked rice
frozen foods tropical fruits and vegetables
milk, whipped cream, yogurt and ice
cream refined oils
hot spices
aromatic
drinks. copper
● {sugar ● alcohol|● alcohol that is
sugar} processed foods. chemical

preservatives drugs and most medicines
29
21

that if we eat only sweets, we will physically
{chicky resemble refined sugar|resemble
refined sugar that is chicky}. If we are
tomatoes, we will be soft and not firm. Of
course, it is a naive state, but what is closer
to people than such a comparison?
The basics of macrobiotics include the idea of
what is a yin force and what is a yang force.
These are phenomena with contradictory
burdens.
another tendency
to
expansion
cooling down
moisture
growth
the decay of passivity
diffusivity
yang tendency to
compactness
drying heating
smaller sizes
activity
clustering

density.

fortress

{physical activities:|Body activities that is né}

etc.

in

opposite poles. The classification was made by the Orientals on the basis of food for the human organism. It is not difficult, moreover, according to Po, a person can guess in a short time where he would classify the food that he

just

Drugs and chemicals

Alcohol

Simple sugars, artificial sweeteners

Fruits Oils and other fats

Vegetables

Legumes

Cereals

Movement

s cheeses

rarity

mental activities:

etc.

We can find hundreds of such opposites. Easy time, for example, the optimal state is one that

{has at nou|at that is has} a tendency to grow,

but while maintaining the strength of the pact. There will be too much tendency towards growth, accompanied by a tendency towards softness, fiddliness and licentiousness. We will then talk about the imbalance in the daily yin direction. According to the ideas of O tu, we can work towards such an imbalance in such a way that our diet is both an excess of foods with an in character.

On the contrary, the yang of food will cause a person to be flexible, intractable, stubborn, and his organs will be weak and immobile. Based on this principle, the oriental treatment of food Diseases was created, in the image of which there were {in the foreground signs of Yin|signs that is in the foreground}, they were treated with yang foods and vice versa, diseases with symptoms required treatment with yin foods. We could easily argue that if we combine food else we get a good balance, This is our diet. We eat meat with cabbage, spread the bread with the butter we bought in the pastry shop, we long for the bread, the heaven of sausages. However, such a situation is similar to the statement that the minimum temperature in the room is 25 Celsius.

In order to know what we are talking about, it is necessary to look at the table that expresses the sorting of foods according to

12

Egg

Meat of mammals

Adek includes a number of foods. When we say others, we would have to list everything related to them, from peas to beans to peanuts. seen by people as a nut, but biologists insist- it is a type of legume. Of course, there are also many beans - we haven't seen them in {our regions or|regions that are ours}. And as for the helenina, If we put in the work, he will name her - well over a hundred. Macrobiotic cuisine is detall- nor the amount of raw material used {is not indifferent|indifferent that is not}. For the hunter, it is necessary to add more yin vegetables, someone ko het and for his health needs a {travin jang|jang that is travin}. For example, children {must make sure they eat more food|make sure they eat more food that is they have to} Idospall. Therefore, the recommended doses of food in the poison {don't take recipes too seriously|don't take too seriously that is recipes}. The recipe calls for one carrot and two lettuce leaves. However, it is summer, your boarder {needs food more jin|food more jin that is needs}. You put {pål carrot Beta| carrot that is pål} to the salad. The food will remain unchanged, only you will be the diner's individuality.

ink is with the cooking time. The recommended time is only at, average. Also at this point {you will think|think that is you will}. the gas tap shuts off much earlier than in winter.

13

CEREALS

Cereals are the basis of a macrobiotic diet. Grain licks natural harmony, balance. Cereals, however, contain different {amounts of minerals,|substances that are also amounts of minerals} fat, and protein. That is why the doctor saw certain differences in their effect on humans. Buckwheat is the densest, most yang ninou. It is not in the true sense of the word 1. it only resembles it in its character. Pati meni and ny red-colored. It contains very little fat-3 has a high mineral content and {bike fiber content|bike that is content} is also substantial.

One serving of buckwheat provides the necessary grain {fiber for the whole day|for the whole day that is fiber}. An interesting feature of the routine is that it has a positive effect on the state of the cells. In fairy tales {buckwheat porridge was called|kaše that is buckwheat} a joke. Perhaps precisely because of its very beneficial effect on mental health. Buckwheat is available in the diet section of many supermarkets. In our lands, you enjoyed the greatest popularity in Moravia, where you can reach with {pagan troops|troops that are pagan}. That's why she was called {i tatarka)| tatarka that is i}

At the opposite end, the most common cereal is KU RICE. Especially corn used in cooking, that is, sweet corn, which has a high sugar content. it is more suitable for the summer months. In {our stores mainly canned|stores mainly canned that is ours}. We can usually also buy kuk semolina..

In the middle between these cereals lies RYZE, T he edge of cereals in the world and in macrobiotics. It is the head of two-thirds of

humanity. It contains {in balanced form| balanced that is in} p substances. In Czechoslovakia we use {uncut with the trade name Natural|with the name that is uncut}. It's brown rice. That's why {in the world of Pika|in the world that is in} she eats brown rice or sake k or integral. When the {Far East was penetrated by the west|far penetrated that is east} lization, rice began to be processed by grinding. Dis Named beriberi, a vitamin deficiency disease Unpolished rice contains more fiber, minerals and {vitamins than rice| than that is vitamins} polished..
Between buckwheat and {rice lies millet|lieží that is rice} and rye, MILLET used to be the most common cereal in the Czechs, and the older cereal consumed by the Slavs is evident. In food stores, it is sold ground into a product called extremely {cereal that is healthy}, especially for Dinhe, it's a shame that it practically disappeared from our menu, ZITD we grind mainly into flour. Whole {grains only rarely|only rarely that is grains}. We get rye flour in the store
AND
The

home bread patent, we can {use a flatbread
that is ji, however}.
between rice and corn is OATS, pše
You are coming to shops other than oatmeal
comes that is né flakes} oats. It is an oat
that
grows without nutrition.
It has a slightly sweet taste. Oats were after
a thousand- {diet that is nej|diet that is nej}.
Oatmeal was eaten by non-ancient soldiers,
but it is also the main part of an early
breakfast. we get Special diapers in grocery
stores. is intended for food, the second wheat
product, wheat bran, is a great benefit for
macrobiotic chicken, are wheat flakes, which
are otherwise interested
Germany..
It has long been prepared for consumption
until after- Comps used to be a regular guest
on the table at- We find them in the store under
the numbers indicating macrobiotics, including
1 table scraper. By grinding, we can prepare
completely black from all cereals.
{and it doesn't prevent it|A v that is doesn't
prevent} us from getting into va-
broken down in the amount of raw materials
for one nent {otherwise that is mentioned}.

make it easier, prepare abnins for mugs. Minoa is a regular tea mug, it holds 0.3 liters.
of the previous study of {different kitchens,| kitchens that is different} that for example * can become: the whole science. Let's at least pay attention to those At first, it is necessary that the breed is sufficiently 1921 {we leave it open,|we leave it open} so that the steam escapes - to remove the foam in which the substances that are concentrated
what to do. Then reduce the flame. We cook-lt-in rice, cover it with cold water. We believe that rice, e.g. {for larger collectives,|For collectives that is larger} we will use it after the bottom layer is already cooked and the flammability of the rice will be improved by soaking overnight or finally. We put the rice on the fifth {or in a small|in that is or} dy or in a pan, the dao of which is lightly greased. it is also possible to cook it carefully so that it grains lacquered rice can be used cold in the rose- eh salad, as will be mentioned later.

22

23

Rice Natural

1/2 cup of rice 160-70 01 1 cup of water ●
pinch of salt
Rice cream
1/2 pea of
rice Natural
● 5 cups of water • A pinch of
salt 24

Because Natural rice is unmilled, it is usually quite a lot. That's why we wash it thoroughly beforehand, wash the grains by hand. Cover the rice with water, add salt and bring the water to a boil on a stronger plan so that the rice does not jump. Cook for 45 minutes. Then we put the bu with the lid in {warm to ripen| warm to ripen}. Total preparation time 60 minutes. We want 1 {prepravide s properties|s that are prepravide} more yang, vario in the pressure cooker. We follow the rules for cooking in this dish and the preparation time is 15-20 minutes.

Already the old Cia cooked rice in a thick pot with a heavy lid, similar to today's pressure cooker. D cooking can also be accelerated by soaking rice for several hours before heat treatment. From rice with the properties of more j rice before preparation slightly obst we get rice with the properties of Sometimes

can meet {rice more polluted|more polluted
that is rice}. Then add 1/2 cup more water
and your foam with a ladle
They rub well and {pour water over the roasts|
pour that is roasts}, salt and roll according to
the basic Natural recipe. We cook for so long,
we boil half the water. Pour the cooled rice
over the cloth or folded {gay we squeeze out
the cream|we squeeze out the cream that is
gay}. We serve horáts mainly to people with
digestive problems
The rest of the squeezed rice can be made into
balls or cones and fried in a little fat.
stewed in the oven
and bones"
Wash and mash the rice thoroughly, cover with
water, add salt and let it cook for 5 minutes.
Then cover the pot and put it in the oven
heated to medium temperature the temperature
that is there} where the rice is stewed for about
an hour more.
Cook the rice according to the recipe for the
basic preparation of Natural rice. Spread the
cooked rice on a baking sheet, which we
lightly coat with oil. Dry in an open oven on a
very
{small flame-|flame that is small}. Rice

prepared in this way is suitable in case we are traveling somewhere. Boil it in water for a few minutes or do not heat it over steam, then prepare it for serving. Pre-cooked Natural rice in this way is especially suitable for holidays, if the macrobiotic wants to stick to the diet he is used to.

Natural rice, cooked according to the basic recipe and slightly cooled, is shaped into balls with wet hands. Wrap the balls. in roasted Other seed, which can be found in vegetable or medicinal plant stores, or pharmacies specializing in medicinal plants. The balls can be served warm, if we keep them at the appropriate temperature {in the selected oven| the selected oven that is in}. In Japan, it is customary to take rice balls for a snack, lunch or on trips.

25

Fried rice donuts
1/2 cup rgte. Natural
cup of water 1/2
onion
1 {polévkoud ice peleničné|ice that is polévoud} sprigs of thyme or other chopped greens 1 egg ●olel

perka salt

The procedure is the same as for the prescription. Boiled rice with the addition of fried onions, thyme or green leafy vegetables, or spices add aromatic spices that do not cause a sharp taste. For the consistency of the cones, mix in the egg. I shape the dough and fry it in oil. Even the food is suitable for when we are eating away from home, hot or cold.

Wheat pudding with peas

1/2 cup wheat tice peas

1 blink

1 onion

and a clove of garlic, marjoram, cumin

3 ice whole grain flour (wheat rebo rou 21 ice oil 2 {cups of vegetable|vegetable that is cups} guar

Boiled wheat

1/2 brak food diaper Special 2-2 1/2 a can of water petka soll

{Cook the peas and wheat until soft, add the slices of raw onion, some crayfish, cumin, salt and adjust a little until greased, cover with bechamel made from wheat flour and bake in the oven. under the pan, thicken again mixing the béchamel, heat the contents dry, add the stock, salt and cover the nut|And bake in the oven Preparation of the béchamel Heat the oil in the pan, reduce to a minimum and mix in the oil, stir in the whole grain or grooved mo under the pan, thicken the mixing béchamel again, heat the contents dry , add the stock, salt and cover the peas and cook the wheat until soft, add the raw onion slices, the crayfish, cumin, salt and adjust it a little until it is greased and cover it with a béchamel made from flour}.

Let's leave the wheat {soaked|soaked that are most}. We cook p Like rice, but slightly for about 2 hours. For starters, wheat is harder than rice. Drain the water from the wheat several times in order to

a distinct cereal taste, which {people are not used to|they are not that are people}, as well as unwanted substances that get into the grains during the treatment of wheat or fall from the air. Salt only after water.

alett WHEAT was crushed for food

preparation. we can get the flour in the store under our flour or we can grind it freshly at the townik. It is also possible to sift through sold wheat

the executioner of the finer parts of a woman.

Wholemeal flour is preferred over white flour. However, it has flaws. The main thing is its short shelf life. Due to the fact that the fat from the grain germ goes rancid more easily if it is stored for a long time.

26

27

Porridge from whole grain wheat flour
1/2 cup diaper: or the same {amount
of
Grahamong flour,|Grahamong that is a quantity of flour} event. Another diaper
flour
2 {remin water mugs|water that is mugs}
Sperke sol! chopped vegetables, 1 medium
big that is them}
cibuie,
raisins

,

poppy seeds of your choice for seasoning! kate
Wheat meatloaf
3 {mugs of wheat medium|wheat medium that is mugs}! carrots 2 vest onions. 1/2 cup of oatmeal or whole wheat flour flake or whole wheat flour that is ných}

- marjora
  m 1
  garlic

Fresh wholemeal flour on a dry {pan until it's done} Cover with water, add cumin, cook the salt for about 3/4 hours on a mirand flame!. We mix occasionally. Season the mash with fresh vegetables, foamed onion and sweetened with raisins and ground poppy seeds.

This amount of {raw materials vysta preparation|vysta that is raw materials} wheat meatloaf t for 4 people. We don't make him a meatloaf in a smaller one. Boiled wheat and carrots un in a meat grinder. We grind one chopped and fried and {raw that is onion} mass, season it with major garlic and salt, thicken the whole grain musk with oatmeal as desired. Mix well, form a cone and bake in the oven at medium temperature for 1/2 hour temperature that is her} hours. Baked sekan with sliced raw vegetables is especially good in combination with a couscous salad, for which
{the recipe will be added later|the recipe will be added later}. Z t Ize also fry the
karbanlag in oil
well pancakes
female Tribute
Fry the wholemeal flour in a {dry pan until

brown|a pan that is dry}, cover it with water and let it stand, preferably overnight. Then we add cumin, marjoram, garlic, chopped raw onion or other roots, salt and we prepare a thin dough like for potato pancakes. Heat the oil in a pan, pour it with a ladle. Add enough batter to the pan to form a patty. Similar pancakes can also be baked on a greased baking sheet in the oven. only the dough has to be a little thicker.

28

29

PRAZMA is probably the oldest {someone's ré has undergone heat treatment|passed that is someone's ré} treatment. Sprouted grain is cooked on a hot stove. Itself {sprouted wheat with a well-known dietary supplement|wheat with a well-known dietary supplement that is sprouted}. By sprouting a macaw of unusual quality. Cereals are among the ph biostimulators. Contain a significant amount of vitamins and fats in the healthiest form. Sprouts can be called the elixir of youth without hesitation.

Sprouted bream
food diaper

any quantity

Wash the wheat properly and leave it submerged for 24 hours in a porcelain or glass container. Change the water for 24 hours, wash again and finally drain. bowl. T {we leave at room temperature|at that is we leave} the temperature Sprouts will appear immediately the second d wheat is ready for consumption in 3 days. If we stockpile wheat, then {it will go down|down that is it will go} in the refrigerator. Sometimes germinating wheat is prepared every day to prevent the appearance of mold, but there is no choice but to throw away the food that is before the appearance of mold. The easiest preparation of wheat is to fry it in a pan. Roasting gives it a taste. It is especially suitable for people with healthy teeth.

{oh food é dietních|Oh é that is food} products can be purchased BREEDING OATS, We will thus obtain a grain that

page has no competition. The proteins contained in the complex are closer to the proteins of legumes than to those of other obilains. The fat found in oats, the important lecithin. Mucous protein avenalin på-enzymes excellent for digestion. All this from oats, which was an important {part of the medieval stra|medieval that is part} of the history of oats, the Swiss nutritionist Bircher wrote his famous muesli (raw oatmeal with fruits) is a reminder of his medical successes even

noves

Washed oats {we cook under a lid|we cook under that is}. 2 hours. Tasty, warm, slightly salted, it is served as a side dish to vegetables. or to other foods.

If we add more water, then the cooked Dves will form a jelly after it cools down, which will be added to the mixture! with honey was successfully used to treat digestive problems in Russia. Even for macrobiotics, oats prepared in this way are excellent

breakfast.

flakes variously flavored

wwwgch Fry the oatmeal lightly

on

dry pans so they don't stick so much. We can add 1, dried grain sprouts that {occasionally appear|appear that is occasionally} in the market. After roasting, they get flakes and chips. office taste Then {we will pour the flakes|we will pour that is flakes}. water,

add

dried or fresh fruit and raisins and cook the mixture to the consistency of a watery mash.
Decorate the surface of the cashew with chopped or grated nuts. If we adjust the dish with salt, we add spinach, onion, or diced
{sliced fried radishes|sliced fried radishes}.
30
31

Macrobiotic Cuba
1/2 cup barley
Rrup
1 cup water pinch of soll 11ce peas
And a clove of garlic, a mushroom, chopped
Verstvé
Rye
pancakes
1 cup of finely ground sweet flour 1 cup of weak mella decoction
cumin • blej
I soak the hail in advance for 8 hours. We drain the water, wash it and add salt again and cook it gently with {young peas,|peas that are young} and dried mushrooms, which we soak in the same amount of hail. They will get smbs

{sap in the oven|in that is sap}, hail so get chuf. Rolled grits {slow cereal supplement|cereal that is slow} to give a macrobiotic tallite

We mix the flour, the decoction from the melta, and make {rid that is rid properly|which is rid properly}. Let it sit for about 2 hours. We heat the oil and in the Ižící sieve we spread the dough into the Ivar, which we properly bake into chutnajf pancakes {in a salty treatment|a salty treatment that is in}. The pancakes were baked in the same way on a dry griddle, so try it today. Such anti-leavened bread certainly has health benefits.

We roll CORN COBS especially on summer days when the corn is ripening. For customs purposes, they are sold in countries where this food has cial forks or spikes, into which we

{fix that is kon} on both. It is then easier to hold in the hands. Cuckoo grits are excellent! baby food.

Corn on the cob boiled

1 {kukung klos voda|klos that are kukung} sat Put a fresh ear of corn in salted water and steam. Depending on the size of the ear, the preparation of the meal takes about 15

or

Pour the cornmeal into the boiling water, which is lightly salted beforehand. We cook on a low flame. 20-30 minutes with constant stirring.

We eat polenta warm, oiled with 1 spoon of Juna or Hera.

Adding raisins makes the dish slightly sweet. If we let the cooked polenta cool in the pan, a jelly-like cake is formed, which is easy to turn out. We can cut it with a weak knife. This results in two thinner pancakes that can be eaten for breakfast spread with sugar-free preserves or prepared with naslama.

{canned foods have been appearing for several years now|Canned foods have been appearing for several years} with milled grains. Maize treated in this way has partly and partly the properties of cereal. I will prepare the diu mainly in the summer days.

32

33

Canned
corn 1 can
corn 277
Needle
porridge
1/2 cup of egg yolks 1/2 cup of water ● pinch of salt
Jahelnik

2   {cups of jahel •|jahel that is cups} 6 cups of

water fresh and dried fruit (plums, apples
and pears!
• 2 {bliky ● oil|● that is bliky} •barley stad
We turn out the contents of the can, heat it up
and use the dish prepared with added salt as a
separate dish to other foods. Other times,
corn
vegetable salads or new dishes. A can will
suffice as a side dish for 3
Take and wash the millet with boiling water so
that it has a slightly bitter taste due to the rapid
aging of this grain, or roast it in a pot that is
dry. They get a golden color {Then we pour
the millet, we salt it|then we pour the millet}
and we cook 20-30 ml of what we want to get
Art.
This dish {practically k pravujeme|k that is
practically} for one person the amount
written is enough for 4 people.
Taken over and washed {boiling millet with
water that are boiling millet}. Then millet me
with boiling water and {uvali obtained millet|
obtained that is uvali} porridge in dried or
fresh fruit from egg whites. Prepare the mass
in a greased baking pan and bake in the oven.
Drizzled with Jočný malt, it is tasty even the
next day. This traditional Czech food, of

macrobiotic quality, prepares the
dessert. cubans
pods
metal
slurry
banks
Take the millets, wash them and steam them.
Then we cover them with boiling water, cook
a thick millet porridge, which we thicken with
whole wheat flour before the end of cooking.
Put the finished porridge in the oven for a
while and after about 10 minutes. we cut out a
spoonful of gingerbread from it. Serve the
skubanky sprinkled with ground poppy seeds,
chopped raisins and doused with warm water
to taste. By June.
Poppy contains a large amount of calcium,
which is a mineral that is very necessary for
the body. That is why we partially replace the
missing dairy products with poppy seeds.
Take the buckwheat and wash it. Before the
actual preparation, we can fry the pohankut in a
{dry pan|a pan that is dry}. It depends on the
quality of the food we want to prepare,
whether it should be more yang or yin. If we
pour a large amount of water at once, the
grains will boil. We will be-1; slowly simmer
the

buckwheat in a small amount of water, the grains will remain whole. We cook the buckwheat for about 201 minutes. We serve it warm as an obl nin part of a macrobiotic tallite.

However, we can prepare 1 dough from it, as described below.

the kitchen has an infinite number of options. m consisting of a combination of {different raw materials|raw materials that is different}. e.g. combine with each other or with solids. The basis for combinations remains the one with the least characteristic taste.

34

35

Combined cereals

3 {dily rice Natural 1 all|Natural that is dily rice 1} millet, groats or wheat

If the cooking time of the cereals we are using is the same, it is possible to cook them together. In the opposite case, we prepare the cereal separately and cook it until the last 10 m.

In the same way, we can eat the leftover cereals from the previous ones. Very tasty soups made from a combination of both vegetables and legumes.

Rice with onions and carrots
1/2 cup rgte Natural
1 cup of water
1
medium onion
1
smaller mrkes
• oi
1
seat
Millet on onions
36
1/2 pea of needles
1 1/2 cups water 1 small onion. I also salted a
small carrot
1 teaspoon of oil
Finely chop the onion, into rings and {fry both
in a small amount of oil|fry in a small amount
of oil that is both}. Pour the washed Natural
rice over the prepared vegetables and cover
with cold water so that it soaks the surface of
the rice, and add salt. This is the tasty basis of
macrobiotic plates. Tastier variants are made
by preparing rice with onions and stewed in
the oven according to the recipe.
and carrots
Carrots Mix them together and put them on the

grill. Fry them briefly. Prisy millet, which we previously p boiling water. Add the water that {poifeh jeme k|jeme that is poifeh} to cook this dish in parts so that the vegetables do not float on the surface. Simmer under the lid for 20 minutes
cauliflower
no
tal rice
We also prepare this food for practical reasons for {more people,|people that is more} and therefore we will multiply the amount of raw materials. by the number of diners.
We cook the collected and washed millet in the usual way, but only for 10-15 mmut so that they are {slightly undercooked|undercooked that is lightly}. Raw cauliflower, possibly in small pieces. with chopped leaves, put it in a baking pan, salt it, add soy sauce mixed with the rest of the water. Place the cooked millet on the cauliflower and cover everything with béchamel made from wholemeal flour. Bake in the oven for 15-20 minutes.
Preparation of bechamel
Heat oil in a pan, add whole grain wheat or rice

flour and fry it while constantly stirring. Then pour in the broth and cook for about 15 minutes.

Cook Natural rice according to the basic recipe and set aside. Meanwhile {chop the onion finely|chop the onion that are} and cut it short. fry it in oil in a pan. Then we add thin slices of carrot, which we also briefly fry. Add browned crab meat to the vegetables or fish fillet and

{chopped cabbage leaf|cabbage that is chopped} and mix. Pour the mixture with a dressing prepared from 0.1 1 water and 1/2

{teaspoon of soy sauce|soy sauce that is teaspoon}. This entire heat preparation takes 5- 7 minutes. Let the mixture simmer slightly and then add the cooked rice, which we mix with the vegetables with a wooden spatula. Let it warm up and serve as the basis of a macrobiotic plate. It is a ceremonial preparation of rice.

37

Rice with carrots and young peas
1/2 cup Notural rice

1 cup of water
And a small
onion

1 cheek of the young
heck
1/2 {128 soy sauce|soy sauce that is 128}
● fly
you
are
This version of jo fon menshinh rice with
onions and mekvi. Finely chop the onion and
fry with a small amount of oil, add sliced
carrots and {young peas|peas that are
young}.
We leave it for about 2 minutes and pour the
maine with the amount of water mixed with
soy sauce. Simmer for 5 minutes. We mix the
salted ryt Natural cooked according to the
basic recipe with the vegetables shortly before
serving.
Oatmeal with leeks
1/2 cup oatmeal
flake
• 1 small
sausage
1
181 soybeans
sauces
• 1 cup of water
a slice of velo sara or brynza
• soul

- materidouška, medunk {al according to taste|

according to taste that is al}
We prepare this dish {the habit of several people|more that is the habit} at once, and therefore we multiply the raw materials by the number of leeks into rounds, and its underground white part, then the green part, and put it in the baking pan. Sprinkle the flakes with water mixed {with sžoven sauce| with sžoven sauce}. Add salt only slightly. An interesting flavor is added by the fact that the prepared dish is flavored with some of the aromatic herbs, f motherwort, lemon balm. Place a slice of ove or brynz on top. Bake in a good oven, first under the lid for about 10 minutes and another 10 minutes uncovered. {If there are flakes, we add more water|If we add more water, that is flakes}. We supplement the prepared food with vegetables and fresh sal Then it forms a harmonious dish

pancakes with sauerkraut

hanka

We soak the wheat jerky in water the day before so that formed a relatively dense mass. Leave the sauerkraut in a colander. drain and mix it with the soaked jerky. We usually don't salt the dough anymore, because the cabbage is usually salty enough; if it seems too dry, add a little oil. Form patties about 1 to 1.5 cm thick and bake on a greased baking sheet.

38

39

PASTA

Flour products make up only a small part of cereals, which is consumed by crobiotics. It is indicated that flour should not exceed 20% customs duty. Nevertheless, whole grain pasta adds variety to the macroli diet. The council of people will not tolerate a sudden you in the first stage. Cereals in intact form, as recommended by macrobi, are difficult for some to digest.

You may have a {constant feeling of hunger| feeling that is constant}, a desire for bread, water including bloating and may observe an imbalance. In that case, they may use a larger proportion of pasta than is recommended in macrobiotics. Dumplings can be made in a similar way for more serious diners. Abroad, for example in Yugoslavia, buy whole grain noodles and spaghetti 1 buckwheat dish with the trade name Sobl. Whole grain pasta st ma also do it yourself.

Whole grain pasta
500 g whole wheat flour (or 250 g buckwheat flour and 250 g whole wheat flour} • 1 teaspoon salt! 1/2 cup water • 1 egg
40
The indicated amount of ingredients is for four people.
Gradually add whole flour to the beaten egg and salt. From the resulting dough balls, which are perfectly formed. Work the dough for a long time until it is smooth. Roll balls on a floured roll with a rolling pin. The resulting pancake is slightly thicker than usual for making noodles from {white flour,|flour that is white} Cut the fis into long strips and let it rest for an hour. If we want to {dry pasta|glass that is pasta} it is above the min heat source, otherwise it is immediately boiled in the stand cooker. After cooking, rinse the pasta with cold water. The varus time should be controlled according to the raw materials used and the thickness of the product. Buckwheat is cooked earlier {than ple|ple that is than}
Nina
these are the colors on the painter's palette. In what maite colors will he use, what shape will

he give them and in what way does the artist express his idea. ay we will create on a plate with vegetables. For the garden - dozens of types of vegetables. Each has its own characteristics, an actor, {its influence on a person|its influence on a person}. When one learns
, I am learning the art of preparing this or that vegetable. Macrobiotics is a game with food expanders and states. Therefore, only experience, just like experience, makes an excellent macrobiotic ku-
Femeslnik. If we are to cook for someone, we must We must know when our species needs to relax, when calm and when excitement is appropriate. me to achieve knowledge of the effect of diet. Vegetables are the face of macrobiotic telife. From that vi- is in {vegetables can be complicated|it can be complicated that is vegetables}. But everything has its own harmony. Choosing vegetables will make it easier for us to - Each vegetable grows at a different time. That will be a clue.
Furthermore, we must realize that there is a huge difference between. For example, let's compare a tomato with a carrot knee to a carrot

stick. One type is: the fruit is soft, fleshy, The root is red and fleshy..

fragile. Everything {together tvo harmony|tvo that is together}, We must observe the same on the plate. It is necessary that there are root vegetables as well as shoots, heads and a large variety of growing vegetables.

in macrobiotics we follow the following rules. Vegetables are more yang than {vegetables soft,|soft that is vegetables} Very vegetables have properties to them. Paths of vegetables grow-

yang and {aboveground náté Havky|náté that is aboveground} have an influence on the organism, such as a head of cabbage or a head of kahe - harmonize both influences. We combine vegetables and the colors express the {difference between individual|between that is difference} from- We use vegetables as fresh as possible. as much as possible of natural forces is left, it has to be cut. When slicing, we use moistened protote {dry wood sucks| wood that is dry} juice from vegetables, which-

If we want to create a celebratory plate, we can create shapes that create a delicious impression even for me. The kitchen draws attention to the fact that we also eat with our eyes. in contrast to cereals, we only heat them a few times - {how many minutes|minutes that is how many}. The longest time for preparing vegetables

41

in the macrobiotic diet is 10 minutes. During this time, we bake, cook for a short or long time {in water,|water that is in}, steam, fry, pressure cook, gratinate, and most often briefly fry and then steam, Tels is recommended for daily use.

Let us now explain this most common type of vegetable in oriental cuisine.

Cut the vegetables into the shape of matches, thin plastic or smaller cubes. Heat a saucepan or pan over a low heat. We cover the heated bottom with a thin layer, it is more correct if we only coat the bottom of the pan with oil or if we use a kettle, when preparing a large amount of vegetables, only the amount of oil in the place where the container touches the heated oil is enough. After a while, add water to the greens and simmer. Of course, we can add spices to 1, which will enhance its taste, but not with its {sharpness or saltiness|saltiness that is sharpness or}. If we sprinkle dried sage on hot oil, the kitchen will have a pleasant and healing aroma. that is healing}.

Soy sauce harmonizes the individual used Therefore, in the water, which we pour the vegetables before {dul we give a spoon|we give that is dul} soy sauce.

Oil is necessary for preparation, because by heating it, the high temperature is quickly transferred to the treated oil. The heat causes the pores to quickly draw to the surface {The juice will remain in it|in that is will remain} and it will not penetrate into it at a delay that would lead to boiling. If we wrap it in egg white or cornstarch, it results in more perfect insulation. The oil will also prevent sticking {We will add salt until|we will add that is salt} during stewing, so that there is no more water. We want-11 to proceed very perfectly, to mix the vegetables during preparation. According to the oriental line Individual {raw materials mutually influence|mutually influence that is raw materials}.

First put the yang vegetables on the pan. In addition, celery, parsley, parsnips, radishes.

Gradually add vegetables with yin properties, for example cabbage or kap at the end {seconds of preparation we add|preparation that is seconds} mostly linin, such as string beans or chopped salad..

For macrobiotics, the popularity of nin loading is characteristic. In general, pickled vegetables are referred to as pickles". It is one of nature's ways of preserving biologically valuable vegetables, which humanity has been using for thousands of years. In a macrobiotic diet, an important part of the plate .To a large extent on 42

. We don't add it to the plate {in large quantities|large that is in}- et morsels. For nutrition, ear {amount of vitamin C|vitamin that is amount} and fermento are important. In the macro-hospitable, whether {vitamin C in winter|C that is vitamin in} we obtain fruits th from vegetables grown in the place of {we recognize short loading,|we recognize short loading that is} medium and long. avins.

They differ not only in the length of preparation, but also in the amount of salt. The most salt will be {in the long-|long-term

on- in} foods, and therefore the more yang will

have an effect,
of language, we {could translate|translate that
is we could}. no, warming". Briefly {pickled
food component of the plate|food component
of the plate that is pickled}. Its effect
according to tradition.
another.
{food pickled foods belong|Food foods that is
pickled} those that sound exotic to him.
Subdue the Oriental nations as an example of
an unripe plum. After three years, they have
and are used for {organism stimulation|
organism that is stimulation}. Nabolt and the
Japanese are balf, for example, to the middle
of the river Soybeans are fermented even
longer with {rice or Yaka|or that is rice}, so
Miso paste, its production takes up to five
years. even liquids are produced with the
highest quality Metelka soy sauce by the
world's leading nutritionist pant Ave-
delivered at a lecture in Budapest in that is
nášce} in 1989 fant If the Japanese learned in
Europe how to ser cars or radios and then hit
Europe in these productions, repay them in
the production of Misa, Tamari and dalted
foods. For the sake of your health." we will
describe

long and short pickled vegetables.
aminka will be about wild vegetables.
and thought that our ancestors noticed them
only for better quality vegetables. Today we
know that was not the case. Wild growing
vegetables are ideal- they are vitamint and
biologically {complexes|complexes that is
active}. After Feliček, daisies, nettles,
strawberry and violet pelica, but also other
plants were added to salads and other
dishes.
Spinach was made from nettles, fennel,
merlik, field mustard, fireweed, Macropet
added seriousness to these gifts of nature.
After all, we would find many prescriptions in
Old Czech recipes
macrobiotic diet. Vegetables formed a
necessary part of the diet. However, some
vegetables have disappeared. You eat
potatoes, such as turnips, to the great
detriment of our nation. Oven-dried watercress
was available
{ent throughout|after that is ent} winter.
43

I described the preparation of NITUKE
vegetables vi in the introduction to vegetables.
This or a similar vegetable was used to create

many dishes of oriental cuisine, but it depended on the mind of the master chef.

Vegetables Nituké I
- onions

2 {roses of kolták 1 lice|koltáku that is roses} canned corn

1/2 smaller kohlrabi 1 leaf of lettuce ● oil
- dispute

1 tsp solo sauce
ittee Malzeny
- 0.2 {l of water|water that is 1} bu

On a stronger flame, heat the oil in a pan to a high {heat violently in|violently that is hot} and fry it cut into crescents. After d {minutes, we add the rolls|we add that is minutes} to the boiled two minutes in sl and a spoonful of corn.

Lightly salt and season with a pinch of ginger [We can also use oil in which ginger has been pickled for several weeks and which is available at the U Salvátora store.) While stirring, prepare the vegetables for a minute. Then we add the dressing prepared from water, Malzeny sauces. We stew the vegetables in an open pan for 5 minutes. Add the kohlrabi until soft. In {the last seconds| seconds that are last} we also mix the finely chopped salad. We will smother the liquid as much as we want to make sauces.

and Nituké

II Perm

sky

We wrap {chopped leeks|chopped leeks} in egg white and place them in heated oil. Vegetables quickly. turn over and after two minutes add the beetroot, which. first, boil for a few minutes, and {grate on a coarse|on that is grater} grater.. Lightly salt the vegetables and throw them in. a few sprigs of motherwort. Half of the next two {minutes we water|water that is minutes}. {fried vegetables with water and soy sauce|And soy sauce fried vegetables with water}. When {the liquid starts to boil|it starts that is liquid}, we add the zelf cut into fine strips. Simmer in an {open pan about|a pan that is open} for 4 minutes. Stir occasionally. When serving, decorate the vegetables with a daisy flower.

the preparation of vegetables NITUKE III can be with crobiotic vegetables for the spring season.

In this cookbook, we do not mention the

preparation of meat, here, when cooking in the Nituké way, we can add, for example, 1 piece of crab meat or poultry to the vegetable dish right at the beginning of the preparation. We really need very little to get ma-ho.

nina Nituké III

arastaa ribulood

gasket

Mat snake

kho zelf

Cut the radishes into thin slices and dust them with cornstarch, put them in heated oil, add salt and, after a few minutes of constant stirring, fry them. Immediately after the radishes are fried, add the peanuts and fry for another 2 minutes. Then sprinkle the chopped {garlic shoots and| garlic that are shoots} with chopped onion and cover with a dressing made from soy sauce and water. We add a chopped leaf of Chinese cabbage and mint after the mixture has been steamed for the last minute of preparation. a minute of preparation that is her}.

44

45

In this latest KE greens recipe, we're going to take advantage of the special flavor {provided by chya!|chya that is provided} by caramelized malt. The pumpkin itself m flavor. Such vegetables cannot be mixed with ad Bitches.

Vegetables Nituké IV

- a slice of pumpkin

Hokkaido and {other pumpkin or parison|or that is other pumpkin} a few slices of Brussels sprouts 1/2 cup of cereal

malt subend not {melons • sill| sill that is honeysuckle}

2 {spoons of soy sauce|soy sauce that is spoons}

0.2 water

Finely chopped pumpkin {sauté sharply in| rapidly that is samohneme} oil, add grain malt, which will caramelize slightly. Then honeydew and finely chop the cabbage florets and salt.

Let it fry for a minute, pour off the water and simmer the soy sauce. This takes no more than 10 minutes to prepare

PH preparation {vegetables TEMPURA edible quantity|TEMPURA edible quantity that is vegetables} fat. That's why we eat this modified vegetable livka {supporting the digestion of fats|digestion that is supporting}

that will be mentioned

अ

preparation of tempura, a deep-frying pot with
a temperature
at the same rate as it dropped, is the
temperature. frying. If the dough stays on
the bottom, k, if it rises faster, is too high.
Tempura
you
pin
Mix some wholemeal flour with water to make
a dough. (We have to prepare the buckwheat or
bran flour ourselves {nat shrotovniku, because|
shrotovniku that is nat} is not yet sold in the
store.) Leave the dough. rest in the fridge for
2- 3 hours. Cut the washed vegetables into
suitable shapes, which are slices, circles, rings,
rosettes or elderberry blossoms,...
Pour enough oil into the frying pan to make the
prepared vegetables float. Heat the oil to frying
temperature. Soak the vegetables. into the
prepared thin dough. If the dough does not
hold well on the vegetables, first coat it in
{flour that is dry}. Dip the vegetables in the
oil. using a strainer. The actual frying takes 2-3
minutes.
Of which 2/3 of the stated time. Let the

vegetables fry on one side side that is né} 1/3 on the other side. Let the excess oil drain. that is we will leave it} Although we use a considerable amount of oil to prepare the dish, the tempura vegetables will not be greasy.

Rapid heating and {superficial precipitation| superficial that is precipitation}. the layer of wrapped vegetables prevents the oil from seeping inside. This way of preparing vegetables has a more festive character, we don't do it too often.

18

Tempura vegetable topping
1/3 cup water 1/4 cup soy {Tamari or shogu Spetka sauce|Tamari or shogu Spetka that is sauce} ginger
The mentioned {raw materials we serve|sch that is raw materials} in a bowl, which he scoops up and pours over the dressing. It is possible to use even ré {oriental sauces,| sauces that is oriental}, but it is soy sauce.

Vegetable Donuts
1 cup whole wheat flour, 1/2 cup rolled oats | flake that is theirs}

face of oil
1 central etbule:| etbule that is ní}
1
mrkey
1 cup of water
2 {12 pieces of soy|soy that is 12 pieces}
sauces
Cut the onion into small pieces, finely grate
the carrot, fry the vegetables in {ole, pour a
little| pour that is ole} water. Sauté the greens
and add a little sauce. From whole grain flour,
oatmeal, water flakes that is ných} we make
the dough, let it rest for 3 hours [If we use
yeast, which is explained in the recipe, we will
lighten the dough and it will be dense.)
Roll out the dough on a sheet and thick. On the
upper half of the slice, mark the circle in the
center of the circle with the shaper and prepare
the vegetable filling. We carefully fold the
bottom p of the plate
{and we press the tests with our fingers|And
we press that is with our fingers} with the
filling together. Finally, we cut the individual
cobbles. Bake the donuts on a greased baking
sheet in
{medium heat|low heat that is medium}
Tina steamed

notated

Cut the vegetables into strips, slices or cubes. Lightly salt and let it sit for 15-20 minutes. In the meantime, let's prepare the pot with steamer attachment. Add a little more salt to the water in the pot. If you add a few sachets of aromatic spices to the water, the steamed vegetables will acquire different subtle flavors.

Special dishes designed for this method of dietary cooking are produced abroad. We usually steam vegetables for 20 minutes. If we want to prepare root vegetables or older kohlrabi in this way, we prefer to use a pressure cooker. The required cooking time is then indicated in the brewing instructions. Green and young leaves are steamed for about 3 minutes. When serving, drizzle the vegetables with soy sauce.

other fondues.

Choose the vegetables according to taste and cut them into cubes {about 1X2 cm|1X2 cm about}; divide the cauliflower into florets and cut the radishes or carrots into rounds. Put in a bowl and lightly. we salt. Also {we cut the sheep's cheese|cheese that is sheep} into smaller cubes. In a special container for the preparation of {fondue, we will heat such|we will heat that is fondue} amount of oil so that we can dip the vegetables in it. The container usually stands {in the middle of the table and| the table that is in the middle} guests skewer the vegetables on special forks with a piece of sheep's cheese. Each of the guests prepares vegetables of their own choice. He dips a fork with skewered vegetables and cheese into it of boiling oil for 2 minutes. Zelent-

new

{fondue is served|se that is fondue} with dressing. for tempura vegetables..

48

49

50

Golden pancakes

100-150 g Hokkaido or jing pumpkin {drich dine|dine that is drich}

1 cup whole wheat flour or breadcrumbs

1/2 cup oat flakes siding that is theirs}

1 egg water st

• cal

Nettle

spinach

2 handfuls of young nettle leaves or tips from older çapito mald onions.

1 {clove of garlic •|garlic • that is clove} otel
• soul

The stated amount of raw materials {LAT two persons|two persons that is LAT}.

We grate the pumpkin on a coarse grater and leave it for an hour d to eliminate the excess in which {then we squeeze|we squeeze that is then}. A mixture of flour, flakes, egg, water and {we will make a dough|we will make a dough}, which we will leave to rest for an hour. We mix the breadcrumbs into the toast and form patties about 1 cm thick with a wet hand. They are placed in heated oil. During frying, reduce the flame until the pancakes are cooked. Badges {had a golden color..|golden that are mal}.

Cut the young nettle leaves into fine pieces with a knife. Finely chop the onion and fry in oil. On an onion base potent {young nettle leaves|nettle leaves that is young}. Pour a small amount of water over the salted spinach in which to steam the spinach. Add a small amount of crushed garlic.

Brussels sprout
4-6 heads of cabbage
1 {small onion|onion that is small}

oil

Washed vario cabbage florets 10 minutes. Cut them up, add them to the prepared osmah onions and salt them. The mixture is heated for 2 minutes. The amount of prepared vegetables in relation to the grains depends on whether we want to cook a die yin or a yang character.

or stewed kohlrabi

leaf of Batka

Cut the turnip or kohlrabi bulb with the young leaves into strips {or cubes,|cubes that is or} no thicker than 1/2 cm. Fry them in a small amount of oil and add very little salt. Cover with water and soy sauce dressing. We will stew the vegetables. Before serving, season with chopped {parsley sprigs or watercress|or that is parsley sprigs}.

{stewed anchovies|stewed anchovies that is puky}

Cokankové {cut the pops lengthwise| longitudinally that is pops}, fry them in a very small amount of oil and salt them. Add a little water and simmer gently. Steamed chickpeas au gratin with bechamel sauce are very tasty [see p. 60).

Finak fries

Hetke pinaka

Clean the parsnip root and cut it into chips {2X1X1 cm|cm that is 2X1X1}. Prepared in this way {cook the fries in salted water|cook in salted water that is fries}. Usually about 3 minutes of boiling is enough to keep the parsnip from getting too soft.

Heat the oil in a pan, fry the parsnip fries and place them in a colander {let them drain thoroughly|let them drain thoroughly}.

steamed morels

Cut the white cabbage into thin strips and the carrots into matchsticks. We bring the water under the steamer to a boil, and first put the zelf and then the carrots on the steamer. We cook. steam for about 15 minutes. Mix the vegetables shortly before serving. Carrots give this dish an interesting color and taste. We salt right at the beginning. preparations.

51

Baked onions

3 {small onions|onions that is small}

Pumpkin on a baking sheet

• 3 slices of

agne

Hokkaido or

a different kind of pumpkin
Peel the onion and put it all in the baking dish.
Bake {in the oven dry|in the oven that is in}
or according to the water until softened.
Dobaff lasts around 30 minutes according to
onion.
Cut the pumpkin into thick slices. Salt the
slices on a greased baking sheet. Bake in a
heated oven for 20-30 minutes, baked on a
baking sheet. Together I bake 2 {carrots
sliced with|sliced that is carrots}
{boiled pods|boiled pods that is pods}
ugh or
If we have fresh pods, we remove the fibers
first and then we {cut them into small blocks|
not into small blocks that is cut}. We cook
fresh {pods in|boil that is pods} in salted water
for a period of time. and: 10 minutes. Cut the
canned pods into blocks without {preparation|
preparation that is previous}. Drain the water
from the softened beans, chop the onion and
fry it in oil. Place the pods on top of the onion
and stir for 2 minutes.
The aisime vegetable is suitable for the winter
months of preparation is quite: long, and
therefore we consider the N151ME vegetable

as a vegetable with {yang properties|properties that is yang}.

We eat vegetables

1 onion 1/4 zelf

1 parsnip •1 carrot sul

Cut the onion into strips, cut the parsnip into strips, and cut the carrot into rounds.

Place the layers of vegetables in the greased ceramic thick-walled iron pan in the following order: first the onion, then a layer of parsnips and carrots. Pour water over the vegetables so that the water does not reach the top layer.

Let's cook over a low flame! or dust in the oven gently. Vegetables before {self folding| folding that is my own}. De heat {preparations takes about|träs that is preparations} 45 Alšime vegetables form a complement to the macrobiotic plate along with cereals and legumes.

52

53

SALADS

Macrobiotic salads form a yin component of the diet. Prote for warm summer and autumn days. Because macrobiotics use {our civilized

world|the world that is our civilized}
environment with its own other, they try to
have the relaxing and cooling properties of the
salts by their heat treatment. Vegetables that
have been pickled, such as beets or beetroot,
are also suitable for preparation. There are no
limits to imagination, as is already widely
known with salads.

10

Salads form an integral part of the diet {in
civilized countries|vilified countries that is in}.
From a soft point of view, this good habit can
be understood as an effort to balance {a large
amount of meat|meas that is a large amount}.
The more we eat {food,|vem that is food}, the
more salads made from raw vegetables can be
served as a side dish. Furthermore {the
mentioned salads belong|the salads that is
mentioned} of the dardized (average)
macrobiotic tallite
Blanched cauliflower and radish salad
how many heads of cauliflower 2 {radish
sul|

sul that is radish}
parsley sauce
He prepares each vegetable Cut the vegetables
into small pieces and steam them. Leave the

vegetables in the salted pot for 2 minutes. Mix the steamed vegetables and serve cooled. Blanched salad with celery and broccoli 1 bulb of celery
2 leaves of broccoli
Cut the celery into cubes, leave the broccoli whole KANE separately and scald briefly in water (2-3 minutes). Place the cooled broccoli in the center and cover it with celery
Blanched salad with cabbage and carrots
54
4 leaves of white sell
1 mrkey
Grate the carrot on a coarse grater and cut it into strips. We scald the creations in salted water. Drain the water, let the vegetables cool and serve the rolls cold.
steamed salad
elcd
Onions, carrots and radishes {cut into cubes| cut into cubes that is}. Let's prepare the marinade. of soy sauce, water, oil, finely chopped basil and {teaspoon of apple cider vinegar|apple cider vinegar that is teaspoon}. Just lightly salt the vegetables, put them in a porcelain or glass bowl and cover them with the aforementioned

marinade. We marinate in the cold. 4-6 hours.
Serve the salad on a large salad leaf.
salad with radishes and carrots
We will use rice left over {from the previous day|past that is from}, or cook Natural rice according to the basic recipe and let it cool. Cut the radishes and carrots into cubes and cut each vegetable separately. {we scald in boiling water|We scald in boiling water} (2 minutes)..
Drain the water and the cooled vegetables. cover with a dressing of water, a few drops of lemon juice and soy sauce. Mix with cold
This salad is a macrobiotic meal for a {warm summer!|summer that is warm} early evening. salad with onion and radish
Boil the peas for a short time, finely chop the onion and fenugreek and scald {in boiling salted water|boiling salted water that is in}. After blanching the vegetables, cook the whole grain noodles in the water, rinse them with cold water and mix them with the prepared vegetables. We serve the salad both cold and warm. Noodle salads can be prepared from seasonal vegetables to taste.

55

Parsnip salad
2 sprigs of parsnips
2 tablespoons of green peas 1 carrot.
1 onion lemon two 2 ice
mayonnaise
Cut the parsnip root into small pieces around the edge 1 Boil them {in salted water|salted water that is} for 5 minutes. Drain the water and let the pate cool. Let's briefly boil the gamel and {we finely chop the raw|finely chop that is} We mix all the vegetables according to taste, we add the amount of lemon so that the vegetables are only light.

flour is an excellent addition to pastina salad.
Salad from vegetables, sprouted wheat and soy
2 Fedkvicky izice sprouted diapers .4 tce
canned et rolled soybeans
1 tice of mayonnaise
The recipe for sprouted diaper {indicated in the chapter|in that is indicated} about the preparation Mix whole or canned with blanched t kami cut into cubes Add sprouted diapers, mayonnaise. We serve it with whole bread, especially in springtime.

Instead of soy, we can use legumes, such as boiled fa or lentils.

SCENTED VEGETABLES

Xel

Cut the zelf heads into quarters and cut out the core. Cut zelf that is into thin strips with a knife or on a special breadcrumb. In a larger container and a tub, mix the zelf with solf, cumin, or add an onion cut into crescents. Mix the cabbage properly with your hands and put it in a stoneware, wooden or glass container. Depending on the {size of the container, we push in the cabbage|cabbage that is the size of the container} by stomping on it or in a smaller container by pressing it with considerable force with a fist. We remove the excess water. We place a washed board on the zelf, which we load with a washed stone. The more loaded the cabbage is, the more durable it is. If we do not process the cabbage in such a way that it drains {our own water and pour|water and pour our own} it only with boiled salt water, it is intended only for short-term storage and quick consumption. A bowl of cabbage. let's leave 14 data at room temperature. to ferment and then transfer to a cooler place where we can store it. until spring.

With sauerkraut

Feket Hetkesek

Clean the blou Fedkev or radishes and put them in a glass bowl. Layer sauerkraut on the fedkev, cover with cabbage water and cover. Let it ferment in a cool place. Eat only after 3 days, especially in autumn, as a refreshing salad.

58
57

Pickled vegetable mixture
1/2 head {menst cabbage|cabbage that is menst}
1/2 bulb of medium-sized celery 2 parsley or parsnip roots 1 carrot 2 onions
● dill
1/2 {teaspoon of salt|salt that are teaspoon}
Grate the cleaned vegetables with a coarse grater. Add finely chopped dill Mix everything thoroughly and pour a little water into a stoneware {container is excluded|that is container}, cover with boiled water so that the layer is hidden under the water Cover the loaded vegetables with a cutting board, weigh down with a stone Leave at room temperature The vegetables are possible consumption on the 5th day. To stop further fermentation, place

the container in the cold
{na pickled in soy sauce|Na in soy sauce that is pickled}
cats
Prepare the vegetables by simply heating the radish bulbs, cutting the cabbage into quarters, and dividing the cauliflower into medium-sized florets. big roses that is them}. Before loading the vegetables {steam separately|steam that is separately}. in boiling water for 13 minutes).
Take it out of the water and put it in a stoneware container and cover it with a sauce made from soy sauce so that the vegetables are submerged. Before serving, wash the vegetables. with cold water. We serve it {from the second day|the second that is already from} after preparation in a small amount as a supplement to the macrobiotic plate.
Vegetables pickled in this way can be stored whole
winter.
We can prepare other types of vegetables in the same way, such as RADISHES, CAULIFLOWERS or CERT NA BEET. It is only required during the fermentation process of Pepa process Pepa requires né} according to

temperature and! 14 days. In length on Pidime tastes. Fermentation can be accelerated by adding curd or sauerkraut.

Light radish pickles

1/4 kg of Fedkuicka leaves 1/4 {12 salt|salt that are 12 salt}

Washed radish leaves, pesto without chemical agents, cut into fine strips. Drain the glass container and salt the container and let it stand at room temperature for 2 to 3 days. Rinse the leaves with water first. Fedkviček can be processed into another dish at our discretion.

Pickling vegetables in soy {sauce they have japo|they have that is sauce} is for cold winter days. Since the sauce has significant yang properties, we can expect the grilled vegetables to help us cope with the cold better.

ve pickles

hey wky

Fry quality wheat bran or Natural rice flour in a {dry pan|a pan that is dry}. Then we entrust 3 {cups of water|water that is cups}. with salt.

Roasted bran

mix with salt water to a thick paste. Put a thick layer of bran mash in the earthenware pot and on top of it a thick {layer of vegetables cut into|

cut that is a layer of vegetables} slices or noodles. Place a cloth and a cutting board on top of the vegetables and weigh them down with a stone. Within 14 days, the fermentation process is completed and the vegetables are ready for consumption. We limit further fermentation by placing the container in the refrigerator. If there are any signs of mould, it is necessary to throw away the contents of the pot.

58

59

SAUCES

In Czech cuisine, sauces are almost a regular part of the daily diet. In macrobiotic cuisine, on the other hand, they are prepared only exceptionally. During the preparation of vegetables, in most cases we stew them, the juice of the sauce is created. Exceptionally, if we want to add flavor to fried or steamed vegetables, we make {one of the listed sauces|a sauce that is one of the listed}. Abroad, preparations for a macrobio vegetarian diet are made in pri after dissolution {in water they form|in water that is in} a sauce similar to our kitchen, although 2 growth products are being prepared.

Bechamel sauce

3 1ices of whole grain wheat or rice flour 2 tablespoons of oil 2 {cups of broth/vegetable| broth that is cups}, fish, from legumes) • 501 Pumpkin sauce

1/2 kg Hokkaido pumpkin

1 cup of broth [vegetable, fish, and tuttenin)

Maizena

Heat the oil in a frying pan, reduce the heat and add salt and a spoonful of whole grain flour or rice flour to the warm oil. Increase the flame and heat it while stirring constantly until dry {Then add cold|add that is then} liquid, preferably broth from vegetables, legumes, salt and let it cook for 20 minutes until the sauce thickens.

If {we fry first|we fry that is first} onion and then we will prepare a sauce that will be delicious

2

and

Cut the Hokkaido pumpkin into cubes and {simmer in water|water that is in} t ka. Soft pumpkin {strainer that is strainer}. Add vegetables to fish or legume broth, and cook. Sauce {thousting as needed| according to that is husting} Cornmeal.)

the sauce

mushroom

s play

tho

non

the sauce

poke

odyssey

Dice the fresh edible mushrooms, finely chop the onion and fry in oil, add the mushrooms and simmer. Let the dried mushrooms soak {in water|water that is in} for at least 12 hours. Season with soy milk. the preparation of which is given in the {Juštěnin, salt section|Juštěnin that is section} and chopped basil. Dust the mushrooms with whole wheat flour, cover with water and cook for another 20 minutes.

This sauce has strongly yin properties in macrobiotic terminology, which is why we only cook J on rare occasions.

Cut the onion into small cubes and fry it in oil. K cold. add water to the onion, season with soy sauce and let 1/2 of it {diny cook|cook that is

diny}. Pass everything through a sieve and
serve 1 vegetable with cereals.
60
61

LEGUMES

Legumes form pitol for a very long time in a
macrobiotic diet. After all, they are probably
part of the {vlech world|the world that is
vlech} menu. A slightly unusual amino acid
doomed them to this fate. Amino acids are
the building blocks of wine. A person needs a
complete set of building blocks for his life.
Such files are difficult to find in the plant
world. Legumes, however, have the same
amino acid composition as meat and often
contain more protein than meat from
slaughtered animals. Beans contain around
20% protein, pork 22% and soybeans up to
34%. We see, they are an extremely rich
source of this important part. If we combine
them with cereals, they complement each
other, we don't have to worry about something
in our diet. then,
Since in macrobiotics we limit the consumption
of meat and even omit it, it is necessary to

ensure another source of protein. For China or Japan, this is soy curd Tofu. It is also called soy protein concentrate and does not contain harmful {substances like meat|like meat that is substances}. I mean fat, soll, but also carcinogenic {substances created by frying meat that is substances}. Ize tofu can be prepared in many ways, under meat, it can also be added to salads or soups. It is also easy to digest, which cannot be said for legumes. Soybeans alone can cause certain {digestive discomforts|discomforts that are digestive}. The correct preparation of legumes is very important, as they contain substances that interfere with digestion. Before cooking legumes, you must soak them for a shorter time, lentils need {2-3 hours,|hours that is 2-3}, it is better to soak soybeans for 12-24 hours. I play and play for 8-12 hours. Legumes are also relatively die fit. It is less known that it is solf before the end. It is important to add spices to legumes. Balance of the mentioned indigestible substances. Satuva marjoram is proving itself.

It's a pity that there is a selection of legumes in our stores, so Beans, peas and lentils are found in many varieties

specific shape, size, shape and {mainly properties|properties that is mainly}. there was such an assortment, our diet would become stale

It has been said that the consumption of legumes in macrobiotics does not depend on whether we eat meat or not.

vegetarians, then some legumes or vegetables are on the table daily. The required quantity is 1 to {ve Itice per person|Itice that is ve na} a day. We combine them with cereals - fine them in soups or process them into pomades y are very tasty if we cook them together with grain- Fodle {cooking times these|cooking that is times} two foods easily com- We recommend a combination of 1:5 to 1:10, i.e. to one.

5 to 10 parts of cereals. If we don't cook them as often, the oleaginousness of the legumes will increase. We usually combine rye, rice with beans, rice with lentils, groats with buckwheat and beans, oats with beans, wheat with beans Cocka

ky

Pea pancakes

peas or

The

reference

Cook Natural rice according to the basic recipe. In the second play. of water, boil pre-soaked lentils and saturej. Add salt before the end of preparation. Drain the water from the soft lentils and mix the lentils into the cooked rice.

We soak and dry the peas. Grind the soft peas in a meat grinder, season with marjoram or saturej, cumin and salt. Add wholemeal flour as needed. Before processing, soak the wholemeal flour for at least 2 {hours with water|pour that is hours} so that it forms a thick slurry. Crumbs from hard whole-wheat bread mixed into the ground pea mixture are also a suitable addition.

From the pea dough {we will make small|we will make that are} patties with a thickness of 1/2 cm and fry them in oil. Sprinkle the patties with wholemeal breadcrumbs. {they will be pleasantly crispy|They will be crispy that is pleasantly}.

83

When cooking {lentils can be added|we can add that is lentils} to the water and

vegetables and thus obtain a whole range of
flavors in

Lentils with vegetables
1/2 cup lentils 1/4 bulb
celery
sal water
We soak the lentil and gradually add some
{types of vegetables,|vegetables that are types}
and carrots to it after cooking. I usually use
root nut, which we cook for 10 minutes.
During preparation
we salt.
Boiled {sprouted peas|peas that are sprouted}
1/2 cup of sprouted peas 1 1/2 cup of water
● salt
We soak the whole peas for 24 hours. Drain
the water and leave the peas in a bowl under a
towel or to germinate. In a drier environment,
water the plant daily to prevent the appearance
of mold. Pea
4 days. This way {sprouted peas edible|peas
that are sprouted} can be eaten raw, but it
will taste better when cooked. Cover the peas
with water and cook for half as long as is
usual for peas. We add salt before
preparation.
SOY BEANS are more difficult to digest and
have other properties. That is why they are
{recommended only|just that is recommended}
for consumption in the summer. For the same

reason, they recommend cooking with {roots of different herbs|various herbs that is roots}.
Roots and soybeans balance their yin properties with their salt content
We cook the soy in a pressure cooker, because it would take 4 several hours to cook it the Klak way. We're going to be in pressurized water {at least an hour|an hour that is at least}.
This time is necessary not only to cook the beans, but also to remove the substance that the beans contain, which prevents the activity of the digestive enzyme trypsin. 6 is combined with oil or with protein concentrates such as meat or eggs. Soy itself is considerable, and the mentioned substance, which suppresses the function of the digestive enzyme, facilitates the absorption of proteins.
boiled
beans
desk
milk
bob
We soak soybeans for at least 12 hours, but they often need to be soaked longer if they are dried. Drain the water. Put them in a pressure cooker and cook them for at least an

hour together with the roots of burdock,
dandelion

or fennel and a spoonful of {soy sauce|sauce that is soy}. After boiling, we drain the water from the soy and use it, for example, to prepare

{soup or sauce|or that is soup}, because it is a broth made from valuable soybeans, soy sauce and herb roots. Cold soybeans {we combine beans with|we combine that is beans} with other ingredients when preparing various salads and other dishes.

About 1/2 of soy milk is obtained from 1 kg of {soybeans|beans that are soy}. Soybeans {soak the beans at least|soak that is beans} for 12 hours.. The next day we put them in a blender, cover with water and blend. Cook the resulting Hdka porridge on a low flame for about 5 minutes. After it cools down, filter the mash through a cloth or {folded gauze|folded that are several times}. It is practical to stretch the canvas. through a colander. The liquid that flows through the cloth is soy milk, which we collect in a container under a colander. We use the obtained milk mainly in sauces (map?. mushroom), porridges and wherever we could use cow's milk. We would have to flavor this milk to drink.

made milk from soybeans will remain

unprocessed, and in macrobiotic cooking we try to process Asti food, we do not even throw away the scraps, which are called ARA. We can use the resulting milk to prepare the porridge. 5 Milk will make the porridge tastier.

64

65

F

green

Soybean

grits

dr from 1 kg of soybeans

salt

1 egg white

• oil

Wha

t

• water

You

be

No

XER

ru

ki

Z

I

Fi
b
o

21
ki
C
r
SI
0
8
04

Pour enough water over the crumble so that the level is at least above the crumble. Lightly salt. Simmer gently for 30 minutes. Top up as needed. We can add soy milk and boil it until the consistency of porridge. Season the ok tali with a smała c Soybean grits can also be used

{in other porridges or|or in other porridges} to make cakes or flatbreads. Ch neutral and {contains many|many that is contains}

We make TOFU cottage cheese from soy milk, which we heat and curdle. If we use warmer milk, the tofu will have a stiffer consistency. Warm milk as! 70 I put for tofu Fiji. For the precipitation of milk, milk is suitable, which is used in dairies to produce tvaro, but it is difficult to find. Therefore, we replace the rennet with lemon. Thoughtful macrobiotics have also invented zp to make tofu in a freezer box.

varoh Tofu

ka

mantare

1

For hygienic reasons, heat the soy milk above 80 °C before preparing the tofu itself. Add lemon juice or lemon juice to warm milk and let it sit for 3 minutes. so that the liquid above the precipitated veroh is watery. If not, the siidia was scarce. After 3 minutes, pour the liquid i

with precipitated tofu in a box lined with canvas. Holes in the box allow excess water to drain. Cover the remaining tofu with a cloth, weigh down and store in the refrigerator. As soon as the tofu is sufficiently tubelike, usually on the second day, we take out the cloth with the tofu and the cube from the box. we immerse the fofu in cold water, in which we also store it.. If we have the opportunity to prepare tofu. in the freezer, let's heat it up first. soy milk at 80 °C. After cooling, pour them into a plastic container and freeze. After freezing, take the container out of the freezer, thaw it and once again let it freeze. In this way, the milk is precipitated and after thawing it becomes jelly-like. a substance called tofu. Usually once frozen food is not refrozen after

thawing, but
in this case, if after melting the mass we
immediately {freeze it again,|we freeze that
is again} we can make an exception.
Soybeans {soak the beans for|soak that is
beans} for 48 hours. We change the water
after 24 hours. Be careful, the beans will
greatly increase their volume. Remove the
skin from the swollen beans, put them on a
baking sheet and put them in a heated oven.
Roast them for about 20-30 minutes. Take the
tray out of the oven just before the beans. they
dry and harden.
67

To make tofu from soy flour, you need to
adjust the pH so that the flour is not old,
because due to the high fat content, it easily
goes rancid. The quality is easily surpassed
by chemistry. The easiest and fastest way is
to prepare jojoba flour in a pressure cooker.
Soy flour tofu
a cup of
water
2 {cups of salt flour|salt flour that is cups}
11/2 Ry siidla calcium sulfate. or
magnesium soil;

or 3 tablespoons of lemon juice
Put the water in a pressure cooker and {pour in the soy sauce. Mix the sifidio or citro juice into the mixture and pour it into the pot, Hr me, heat at full pressure for 7 minutes. Then we leave the container to cool down slowly. A whey will form inside the toy, which we pour onto a tofu-lined plate. Let the liquid drain, cover with a cloth, put it in the cold and let it harden.

Tofu made from soybean flour has different {properties than tofu from whole soybeans|tofu from whole soybeans that is properties than}. Above all, grit. Therefore, it is more nutritious, but digestible. We should use it only after heat treatment. Raw tofu is mainly used in salad dressings.

AZANKS

addition of our nation, bread occupies its fixed and in this chapter the problem of what to do with bread, if at butter, lard, sausages.

we can use any leftovers of vegetables for spreads. They also do not fantasize about the use of individual species. Therefore, take the above. as a source of inspiration.

nka from Roman peas (chickpeas)

we

ski

Boil the peas and grind them in a blender or sieve them. Salt and {mix with finely|with that are mixed} grated onion! and chopped chives. We present this spread because it is very tasty and in Asian countries. {is called by the appropriate name humus"|With the appropriate name humus" that is called}. Chickpea used to be a very popular legume in our country.

new spread

to

Fry the chopped onion, finely grated carrot and {chopped cauliflower|cauliflower that is chopped} in a little oil. Next, let's prepare the Angch {thick salty flaky|flaky thick salty} porridge. Mix the fried vegetables with the mash. If we want to make the spread more delicate, we simmer the vegetables for 3-5 minutes and eat the pasta. Instead of the flaky porridge, we can also use Natural rice cream.

Sprinkle the spread with fresh chopped nati.

nat et

vegetable spread

erak

at 1
Let's prepare a vegetable spread - 1 cu. Grease
the fireproof mold with oil and fill it with the
prepared mixture. Close the mold with a lid
and bake at 180 °C for 1 hour.
69

70
Bean and pumpkin spread
14 cups of jazoll • a slice of Hokkaido pumpkin
12 {18 cups of soy sauce|soy that is 18 cups}
● satureik
a 1
onion
• oil
We cook the beans with botnym sp saturejka
and soll. The dhame were really soft. D on the
fried onion, mix the Uvat, or a meat grinder
and add the pumpkin and mix with the sauce.
For greater subtleties, if we work the spread
further with a spatula, the chefs use a special
grooved bowl for this, the beans will spread
the wooden
EVKA
must be a completely regular part of the
macrobiotic- Against our traditional soups,
they have several Vari with a short time, 5

10 minutes. Sky too. pant Rettigová drugged the Czech ladies and girls, fathers are not used. the world is the basis of {soup broth|broth that is soup}. Popular foods include many purines that are not good for you and {kidneys here are the best|kidneys are the best here}. That's why otika prefers to use! broths from other foods.

He didn't-

seaweed is used to prepare the broth. They didn't tell you about the races, because they are not on the shelves {we only get them|we get that is ours} in the shops of medicinal herbs.

There we can buy bubble kelp and From the Soviet Union {imports canned| imports that is se} desolate, Meeralgen is

available. The mineral content of these gifts of the sea is admirable. Not long ago, a factor affecting people's condition was discovered in Pasá - In order to orient ourselves correctly in Lasas, we had to! to learn their foreign-sounding names, for example or, wakame, hiziki or arame. They say you have it in you. pamer of the elements because they come from the sea, just as we make a broth from them by boiling them {in water for a time|in water for a time that is in}. 60 minutes.

{fastou components of soups are|fastou soups that is components} mushrooms. In oriental use it! with the likes of wood rot fungi. Even in those cases, a factor that has a favorable effect on blood vessels, foreign mushrooms will be replaced by our boletus or oyster mushrooms, however, wood-decaying mushrooms have already appeared in organic stores.

Live {we balance the raw materials with soy| we balance that is raw materials} with sauce or pas- Mn Soups have a little more macrobiotics in their prime - hu than here. Do not eat before the main meal, because- tivact States that {we need to spend|we need to spend that is necessarily}. either as a separate meal or with a thin jidio soup.

soups from winter soups Its tim that vegetables me in larger pieces. We also use more root vegetables, more soy sauce and oil.

71

Summer soup
* 1 mrkey
1 stalk of cauliflower 2 l of green peas
and onion
a few stk trocele a few kolika {violet tricolor

1/2|tricolor that is violet} lb solo sauce naté patitky or {Other green naté|naté that is

other green}
Winter soup
1 slice of celery
• 1 parsley • 1/2 kohlrabi
• 2-3 {stems of cabbage|stems that are stems} 1/2 onion
801 oil
1/2 teaspoon of soy sauce, a handful of oatmeal flake that is theirs}
stewed vegetables

We clean the vegetables, cut them into smaller pieces and stew them in a small amount of water, add 1 liter of water or finely chopped {wild herb leaves|wild herb that is leaves}.
Cook for another 5 and 27 minutes. At the end of the cooking time, add soy sauce. Sprinkle st nati.

We clean the vegetables, cut them, cook them and lightly fry them in a large amount of oil.
Pour 1 liter of water or broth with soy and soy sauce and add salt. Winter soup with {more than summer soup|than summer soup that is more}. Add a handful of oats to thicken the soup. About 7 to 10 minutes. Dried nate {soak

before giving|giving that is before} and season the soup.
Wild herb soup
{several young leaves of pampeiia|Several leaves that are young}, itrocele, contryhele, poppavy,
mochny hust (choose with {depending on the size of two|size of that is according to} types 2-3 dandelion roots and topucha kittens •1 small onion ●otel
with
a handful of oat flakes vioček that is ných}
• soy
sauce
72
Coat the bottom of the heated pot with olive oil and place finely {chopped onion|onion that is chopped} on top. Fry for a short time and cut the fresh or dried roots of dandelion or burdock into rounds and add to them. Pour in 1 liter of water, throw in a handful of oven flakes, salt and cook 10 Before the end of boiling, add a few drops of soy sauce.
from beans and sauerkraut
Jason
celery
nice
131

We cook the beans {in a larger amount|in larger that is in} water, so that we don't get a thick mush after boiling it. Towards the end of cooking, about the last 15 minutes, add sauerkraut, diced celery and oatmeal or sprouted beans to the beans. or that is né flakes} wheat. Season with marjoram. The soup is also excellent the next day.

tallow soup

y marine X3 cm

mushrooms

Athene hehe

ground

or according to

We prepare an oriental soup for four people. In {our conditions|the conditions that are ours}, the easiest way to get agar-agar, bublenatka or sea cabbage from the Soviet Union is from sea fas. We cook the sea goose together with the ginger root. If we don't have dried ginger, we use ground ginger. We add dried mushrooms to the broth, which we previously soaked for two hours. We have to cook the mushrooms for 15 minutes. And 10 minutes {before the end of the boil|at the end of that is before} put the muggle into the broth, add soy sauce and add salt. For the last few minutes, let the tofu, cut into cubes, cook in the soup. If we pour the soup. into bowls made of fish porcelain and light a fragrant offering stick, the illusion of Ortent will be perfect.

73

BREAD

Bread baking is {several thousand years old| several thousand years that is old}. Bread is baked in Europe: the ancient Greeks. This bread certainly did not look like a bakery product. It was a mixture of wheat and rye flour. Gradually, bread and other types of cereals were consumed, mainly barley and rye, but also corn bread. In many {countries the bread represented|chléb that is zemich} rather different thick plackoa Vie pechen in the oven or on a plate stove, rarely on k In Czechoslovakia, bread flour is milled ser wheat and bread dough is prepared kynutin Macrobiotics hears his dining room, but doesn't like to see him there. According to macro rules, bread has {jong properties| properties that are jong}. It contains salt and long-term baking is not a food preparation in macrobiotics.

Macrobiotics are not put on par with the yeast from which yeast is made. Omerit mact bread, however, means to grow with a habit and with porridge, and this is the prerogative of aged bacrobiotics.

The pH of bread preparation depends very much on the ingredients from which it is made. Essentially, technology that combines grains with wholemeal flour must be used all over the world. Also, the freshness of the mooky influence. The quality of the taste of the bread can be improved by adding sprouts, sunflower seeds or sesame.

the wine industry is in any case many healthy, modern foods. More commonly, only whole grain breads such as graham or ki and Kiev bread. That is very little. That's why sit {asto whole grain bread bake semi|bread bake semi that is asto whole grain}.

yeast
{lini 2itné flour|Lini muky that is 2itné}
larn wheat flour or
no flour and 300 g whole wheat flour
**** yeast
mix a handful of flour with a little water and make a long dough. We wrap it in a damp

cloth, place it in a porcelain or earthenware
container and {let it rest at room temperature;|
let it rest at room temperature}
moisten it slightly, but do not do anything with
the dough; Add 12 cups of flour and a little
water. We work everything thoroughly and
wrap it again in a scarf. During the day we
will still work lightly;
we ascend as on the third day;
procedure same as the third
day;
kvasek botov and we can start making bread.
{ayt we leave a little leaven|Ayt we leave a
little that is} directly and inoculate. the next
dose, the process goes faster. After a certain
but the yeast culture becomes old and the
bread ceases.
and bread
500 g of flour, preferably freshly ground. He
shared the rye
of flour can be quite large. Rye bread is chutt,
in the Czech Republic we give {usually
smaller dil|smaller that are usually} t- Mix the
flour with salt and cumin, add quark, promise.
We add water so that it works well. We
process the dough for about 10 minutes, then
{form it into bread,|form that bread with it}
Place the bread

carefully on an oiled baking sheet, cover with a towel and let it rise for 2 to 4 hours. No process takes place in the morning hours. The higher the temperature, the faster the bread will rise.
When they are added to the dough, the hole must not level out quickly, so that the bread rises. We heat the oven to 200 al 0 and bake the proofed bread for about one hour. Into a bowl of water so that the environment preserves the primer bone.
Rice bread belongs to the category of less tasty, thicker breads. We can prepare it with sourdough. When we are going to bake bread without leaven, bond) of grain that was cooked a few days ago, protal 1

Rice bread

3 cups whole wheat flour one cup mate gt other flours) 2 12 soll 12 cups kedsku • 2 cups water {4 peas boiled|boiled that is 4 peas}.
{rate Natural olet|Rate olet that is natural} Oshawa bread
2 1/2 cups whole wheat diaper flour
112 gram flour

a cup of rice flour

12 {soll teaspoons 5|soll that is teaspoons}
drops of oil

2 {pody mugs|pody that is mugs}
All {we feel the raw materials thoroughly with
our hands|we feel thoroughly with our hands
that is raw materials}. The dough is sticky, so
we sprinkle flour after. Put the dough in a
mold with oil and leave it to rise. We bake for
hours in the {form that is in the form} in an
oven heated to 250 °C. If the yeast is not
active, let the dough rest for 24 hours. During
that time, you will {we will add another cup|
we will add that is} flour.

First, we mix all the ingredients. Then we add
the oil. Gradually add water and knead. It can
be a little thinner {than for shortbread|for
shortbread that is than}. We heat the pel mold,
wipe it with oil, roll the dough into it, and
leave it to sit covered with a damp cloth for
several hours. Bake the bread for 1 hour in the
oven at 200 to 250 {°C warm|warm that is °C}

ERT

and refined sugar, these are two completely
unsmi- This, of course, {does not mean
banning sweet foods|banning sweet foods
that

is does not mean}. to obtain a sweet taste from sources other than kr. At the beginning of macrobiotics, it is therefore necessary to get used to sweet foods with sugar. There are some precautions for this. First of all, reduce consumption. These are Yang foods, which on the basis of {pra plementarity:|plementarity that is pra} attract a person to yin foods!-Often to easily available sugar..

the abdohl of switching to a macrobiotic diet is arat barley malt. It is made from sprouted liver, wort is boiled and by thickening it hs, malt syrup. Many countries produce this sl-love.

For example under the name Biomalz.

we eat sweeteners that we know from history. Maturely. {main dried fruit|Main fruit that is dried}. At the world food exhibition in 1989 in Paris, Nestara pracharanda created a sensation with crushed dried pears. we, of course, take it there, but others. Nuts are eaten. Roasted lelices are used for desserts that are delicious, such as an apple and grated into it. y den is deliciously sweet..

{The taste of onions is sweet|The taste of that is sweet} and carrots. She grates herself into the dough and sweet carrots are made. raisins are a macrobiotic sweetener.

cake

{Yukuričné Jablečne delete|Yukuričné delete that is Jablečne}

Mara

Corn grits! we mix with apple juice, jam boiled without sugar or barley malt, a pinch of salt and water. Simmer the mixture for at least 1/2 hour on a low flame for coughing. Then we add unburnt grated almonds and {a few drops of lemon juice| drops of lemon juice that is a few}. Make sure the porridge is thick enough. Heat and spread on a greased baking sheet and bake for 15 minutes.

After cooling, the cake will harden.

76

77

Corn pudding.

2 {cups of corn flakes|corn that is cups} CORN FLAKES

● soda

50 g of raisins

2 apples

{a piece of ground roasted vanilla|A piece of ground roasted that is vanilla}

Orishas

Sprinkle the cuckoo flakes. Add ground raisins. poached apples and a piece of vaika Cook for 20 minutes on low {j until that is j} thin porridge pus The indicated amount is enough for the bowls. Moisten the bowls and pour ground roasted {Pl that is nuts into|Pl that is nuts} bowl..

If we use coffee decoction instead of water, a pudding with a coffee flavor will be created. agar-agar

or

agar

ce

We soak the agar-agar strips in water for an hour and then boil them with the fruit for about 5 minutes. Dissolve the agar-agar and pour the obtained mass into bowls. The indicated amount is enough for 4 bowls. After cooling, it solidifies into a firm, jelly-like consistency.

Warm {agar-agar we can grind|we can that is agar-agar} on fruit placed on a rice cake or on a pancake made of whole wheat flour.

pumpkin filling

whole grain

risks

Mix whole wheat flour with water, oil and a

few {grains of salt|salt that are grains}. We will make a pliable dough. Roll out the dough into a patty about 3 mm thick and place it on a greased baking sheet. Pre-bake the pancake in the oven for about 30 minutes. Apples cut into thinner slices and {simmer pumpkin slices| pumpkin that is slices} in a little water, pass them through or. otherwise we grind. This way we get the stuffing, which we layer on the baked flatbread. Sprinkle the edges of the pancake with grated ofifis or nuts. Bake in the oven for about 20 minutes. If we add 2 strands of sourdough leaven from the third {day of production,|production that is day} to the dough, the dough will be lighter. In that case, let the dough {rest for two hours before baking| rest for two hours that is before}.

Hickies from oatmeal wangeh| flake wangeh that is ours}

Points

Mix the flakes, flour, raisins, salt and cinnamon. Add oil and water to the mixture and process. Leave the dough. rest after 1 hour.

Then with your hands. we make patties about 1 cm thick and bake them in the oven until golden. Oatmeal patties are | flocek that is ných} quite durable and can be stored for a long time in a dry place.

79

78

80

Apples with oatmeal
* 1 cup of
oatmeal
pad
3 {mugs of water|water that is mugs} 2 ice cubes of Malzena
raisins
3 Apples
6 orlikd or 3 vtala nuts
Rice cake
3 {boiled rgte mugs|boiled that are mugs}
Natural
* cup of thick flaky kate 50 g raisins •
50 gotska 3 Jabika seasonal fruit •
pie!
Carrot Cookies
2 cups of oatmeal flake that is theirs}
* 2 carrots
1 egg 60 g Hery water.
Lightly fry the flakes in a pan and cover with water. Add raisins, washed chopped grated nuts and cook the porridge. Five minutes

before the end, add cornstarch to the water to make a

porridge. If we have ar, we add it instead of Malzena. VR will be even better. Let the cake cool down, put it in an oiled oven and bake [20-30 minutes].

Cool boiled ry Natu and cold flaky kali walik with washed grated {apples ground raisins| ground raisins that are apples}. We form a 2 cm flat cake with raised edges from the resulting mixture, then bake it in the oven for 15 minutes on a clean baking sheet. Layer the seasoned {ovar cake with chopped ovar nuts| we sprinkle the cake with chopped ovar nuts that is ovar} nuts on the baked pancake. If we use vests, cover them with ground mace boiled with raisins.

Grind the oatmeal {ve srot ku|srot that is ve} into flour. Grate the cleaned mrkes on a fine grater {struhas add eggs|add that is struhas}, Hera and se and mix with water. We will work out a stiff dough, which we will leave to odish as! 1 hour and then turn it into a pancake. Cut cookies from the pancake with a cutter, which we bake on a baking sheet for: 30 to 40 minutes. Upe {biscuits we can glue together| we can that is biscuits} jams prepared without sugar.

TAN
the prescription of the macrobiotic cookbook will be obláma under the name SEITAN. The raw material for the product is actually grain gluten, which can be bought at local stores.

Under the name grain meat.
for example, a store of {rational nutrition in| nutrition that is rational} Hello. It is a protein concentrate. We mentioned that
it recognizes only complete foods, but it goes beyond the symbolic meaning of the word meat. This only represents food, but there is 1 symbol in it
wealth, enjoyment and dominion over nature. it is not only a physical issue, but also a psychological one. acrobiotics had to invent meat.
en (grain
meat)
wow
Moka
Mark
let's go
Mix coarse wheat flour with water to make a dough. Immerse the dough in cold water and

{let it rest for an hour|rest that is let},
possibly all night. The longer the dough is
immersed in

water, the easier the next preparation is. After it has rested, we start washing the starch out of the dough. We wash it under water and change the water as long as it is cloudy. A good improvement suggestion is to place a bowl in the sink and {let it flow slowly|slowly that is let} the water, which will wash away 1 starch as it overflows the rim. After the starch is washed away, a spongy mass is formed, which {is named|is named} coffee.

we prepare it by taking 3 parts of coffee and one d {not flour,|flour that is not} water, salt and a reasonable amount of soy Vie mix, thoroughly knead the dough into balls, rollers or a long snake. Prepare water with dates, like when we cook dumplings. Add the ostrich sauce, celery, onion and ginger. Boil the water and put the dough in it. Seitan acquires a varén.

, that's why we count on it in advance. In an ordinary pot. tan 1 1/2 hours, in pressure 1 hour. Let the liquid cool, it can be used as an excellent and nutritious soup. Seitan

81

we will make it in stock. We keep it in cold

water. If we change the water regularly, drain it 14 dat M blotici eat soltan no more than twice a week, Homage as with meat. PM its modification we can visit sy classic cuisine. If we chop it into cubes and simmer it, we get a {delicious stew|a stew that is tasty}.

with

Baked seitan is made by putting the solan {cut into slices|on that is cut} into a fireproof dish and covering it with elle nekem and sprinkling it with thyme. Add 12 cups of soy sauce, cover with half a cup of water and cook in a covered dish in the oven for 45 minutes. We prepare settan riskies by rolling the slices in flour, eggs and breadcrumbs and frying them. We can come up with hundreds of ideas.

We can use it to pre-treat meat from any cookbook. Seitan is served with vegetables and grains so as not to violate the Ja-Jang pem. They are the meaning of this entire cookbook.

AVER

Macrobiotic day

over the years, ok learns to monitor the reactions of his . Learn with self-diagnosis.

Information for him is: mental feelings, mood, as well as unpleasant boa-ad, anava or swollen eyelids. They manage their food accordingly.. they try to respect the rhythm of their or- I nature as much as possible, they follow a certain time schedule for eating.. a little later than is customary here. According to the biological clock, the stomach is not in optimal shape until around eight o'clock. The composition of breakfast is an important thing.

If we eat mains, eggs and similar foods of a yang character and many minerals, we will soon feel hungry. at the point of complementarity, our body begins to attract pet foods. That's why we long for a snack, {often tvo-sdkostmi|tvo-sdkostmi often}. This creates a habit, the organism gets used to it requires the satisfaction of his habit. The macrobiotic in the day must have a yin character, i.e. a relaxing effect. The start will be better if we are in a relaxed, calm mood. decomposing {starches will ensure a sufficient| ensures that is starches} dose to our bloodstream and we will calmly endure until In the human gene pool, breakfast will not be too deep. I'd say it {will only be a few|a few will only be} a hundred years. and is composed mostly of a watery obtained mash, with an

appetizing taste. To this day, the Chinese eat boiled, unpickled vegetables for breakfast. According to the Orientals, pickled vegetables adjust the activity of the liver and translate well tra are said to be an organ I ensure a good mood.. lant we drink cereal coffee, which according to our Pist blood. Those who like tea will make herbal tea. Beth Strawberry, raspberry and blackberry acidified with Mpku fruits or lemon for sure
I will drink. There is Javorina tea or herbal tea on the market.
the macrobiotic is prepared from the basic macrobiotic rota. He will make sure that it is only light and not burdensome- argantemus. It is useless to exhaust yourself by digesting fats of proteins. A macrobiotic sandwich or soup
{or legume soup|legume that is or} will provide the necessary energy!! afternoon. Macrobiotics drink water for lunch, and a glass of beer.

82

83

Dinner is the richest meal of the day. It has its own function and prepares the organism for cold and vlakos Budg-11 1st macrobiotic as

sparingly as I recommend, they must have {fear of obesity|of obesity that is fear}. Dinner is the daily meal, to the most yang character. A complete macrobiotic diet is ideal. At dinner, it also appears on the plate {most often Dinner provides energy|Dinner that is most often provides} for the person's activities for the rest of the day. We recommend eating no later than three hours before
by that.

Macrobiotic year

Life takes place in many periods. The basic period is d The middle cycle is a year and the longest is a life. In the year pl goes through four periods in which four times ph does not. However, modern man pretends not to see this.

Just put on a thicker coat or go on vacation. Because man lived in harmony with nature for millions of years, his nism still honors its rhythm. If the rhythm of nature follows me, the consequences do not appear immediately, but only after years of fatigue, a decrease in resistance.

di

The annual cycle begins in spring. The liver was considered the basic organ of this period.

After winter they lack mines, they are overloaded with a large amount of salt: and fat. Its the most critical period of the whole year. People commit the most suicides, the weakest children are born, and the most die in the face of this crisis during the Spring Fasts. It meant that it was not safe to cleanse the body with blood-purifying teas. Not even today! such a throw away. A person can help his liver in the spring by consuming all the nati that come from the earth. the macrobiotic flora consists predominantly of leek, watercress, garlic, dandelion leaves, and nettle. This and flax are healthier than greenhouse salads grown with a screen of artificial fertilizers. Because everything that germinates, remember, allows the macrobiotic to germinate to the maximum extent, even legumes. He finishes his pickled vegetables, goes outside a lot, breathes deeply.
Citi, That his powers are returning. He's off to a good start and won't be sick all year. 1 is looking for energy in the sun.
In the summer, it is hot and the roof circulation is the most loaded, m heart pain is obony. It must be extinguished with the first fire, which is usually strawberries. Carrots, kuku raw

salads come to the fore. Meat, which greatly burdens the circulation, is reduced to a minimum. Light oils are used in food, such as soybean oil or other vegetable oil with a yin character. In sub

84

suitable glass of carrot juice and {seasonal fruit|fruit that is seasonal}. Have z {beetroot has a great dietetic effect|has a great dietetic effect that is beetroot}.

it is a time for depressed moods. People are {threatened by the way|they threaten the way that is}. That is why we pay extra attention to exercise that is nat. Deira function of the large intestine will protect us from inflammations of the respiratory system. With {the cold coming on|the cold that is coming on} the consumption of animal protein, which is necessary for the digestion of fiber. Therefore, we will take care of the abundance of {dietary fiber|diet that is fiber}. The main vegetables of autumn are zelf and cabbage. oriental doctors designate the more desirable cereal of autumn worry equinox! begins with the holiday season. People se da, 2 merrily. A person drinks more, more spices, because he wants his own. Winter was considered a bad season for That is why the oriental doctor {recommended legumes,|legumes that is recommended} What is the medicine for this organ. Root vegetables and brussels sprouts, medium {long-seasoned vegetables,|vegetables that are long-seasoned} are caltbrs in a fight with the unpleasant winter depression at pant. Of the cereals, it is mainly buckwheat. So the year will burn out, and it will repay us with the fact that we will be able to call many such things in our lives happy.

Macrobiotic life

vot is the longest cycle a person can go through. divided into a series of smaller and even smaller cycles..|cycles. that is smaller} wykle we divide our life into the period of childhood, adulthood MAM. Each period has its specific features, and therefore the period requires {a certain approach|an approach that is certain}. An adult person is already what {has a taste|a taste that is has}. It is possible to gradually introduce the child to whole grains and vegetables. Teach me even that, Bivot, success in life will depend on how much he can control his life. This leads to {cestal a reasonable diet|reasonable that are cestal}.

Yasina children {need quite high|relatively that is need} doses of protein ket growth and building of nerve tissue. Some of these proteins should be of animal origin. Pin? This will still be the subject of investigation. Then enough to prevent growth retardation, signs of poor development, mental retardation and, on the other hand, that the child should be beautiful, shapely, lively, but it is {sometimes difficult|difficult that is sometimes} to please two masters. sleepiness decreases the need for animal protein, especially work without {great physical load does not require a rich diet|load does not require a rich diet that is great physical}. Also, many non-mool, body 1 du- require a regimen that closely resembles macrobiotics.

25

A number of adults also turn to mike biotics for spiritual reasons. If he chooses a reasonable transition from the usual st to study the laws of macrobiotic life, there is no danger. On the contrary. They will gain an extraordinary knowledge of themselves and their surroundings. Some people are in danger.

Excessive weight loss and anemia These are signals that it is necessary to increase the supply of livestock metals.

A person at an older age does not have such great demands on animal {proteins|such great demands that is proteins}. Fish and poultry fully satisfy his needs. Whole grain cereals must be chosen wisely, because of the stump damage {his digestive tube tends to be different|the tube tends to be different that is his digestive}. However, Nike will not harm the movement that macrobiotics promotes not breathing exercises at all. Macrobiotics is also a kind of vanguard in the fight for food, the biological cultivation of food, its gentle care. Many organizations are {not happy|they don't have the joy that is}. I am sure that if everyone sweeps in front of their doorstep, when we don't care about our personal ecology, we won't have to worry about keeping ecological principles in our whole country.

Tables of occurrence of selected elements in foods

CALCIUM

need
developing countries developed countries
tlin sources of calcium
400-804 mg 800-1000 mg
88
lactating 2,000
mg mg/100 g
mg/100 g
16.
Hiziki
1400
114
Combo
8001
3
Wakame
1300
20
Crazy
260
yoves
55
Aram
1170
flakes
53

Kelp
109
3
32
Dulce
587
22
dried marjoram
1388
38
{parsley nat dried|parsley dried that is nat}
972
139.
nettle
dioecious 57
dried
372
59
groin goat leg
504
228
mochna husf
493
150
primrose of spring
103
(primrose)

722
128
fresh chives
325
76
{dried celery stalk|Dried celery that is stalk}
1,615
1400
dried dill
135
124
ground paprika
239
outlines
93
vanilla.
482
nuts
37
cinnamon
1436
your seeds
1180
seasoning
card 837
fresh chestnuts

38

bean pods

59

seed

s 51

who

46

no seeds

120

zell

45

138 parsley {nat fresh|fresh that is nat}

193

A flour A Pasa aager

59

pore

55

radish

108

400

spinach

57

bubbly

1200

cabbage

92

87

sauerkraut

46

wild mustard

leaves 5.0

nat radish

119

hen pastus!

{dried celery nat|Dried celery that is nat}

6.4

12.0

broccoli

103

capsule

dried dill

2.2

2.2

on chard

203

raisins

ground

paprika

35.0

dandelion leaves

Orthic

1.7

187

dried rose
hips
vanilla
53.3
savoy cabbage
179
fresh raspberries
and nuts
0.94
cinnamon
17.25
your seeds
10.5
kotenf curry
75.0
Animal sources of calcium
e chestnuts fresh 0.75
seeds bean pods
1.0
11.2
zell
2.76
ic seeds
7.1
Brussels sprouts
0.91
carrot 3.5

0.641
Goat milk
150
sardines
you
flour
19.2
a shoe
8.0
cow milk
112
lean beef
ha Pasa
sheep's milk
180
por
k
gar
5
parsley and fresh radish
4.3
1.81
yoghurt
180
(diameter
) bubbly
8.7
spinach

2.1
brynza
844
tourist salami
29
Chinese zelf
0.72
hard cottage cheese
152
rabbit
13
sauerkraut
0.5
cheese Mayor
887
trunk
12
black currant.
1.16
Eidam cheese
669
Hermelin cheese
12
darts
0.81
trout

24
Moravian loaf
cheese 6.3
strawberries.
0.77
herring
29
Olomouc cheese curds
anka dried
374.2
raspberries.
0.9
mackerel
23
fatty cottage cheese 40% 1st c.
left nat dried 22.3
blueberries
0.8
duplex
raisins
2.8
30.64
apple fritters
2.4
Citation: Kajaba, 1. Sarha, O.: Tables of
composition and {values of edibles|values
of

edibles that is worth}. Merkur, Prague 1988. Alain Saury: Les algues, source de vie, ed, Dangles 1962. Richard Mabey: Food for free, ed. Fontana/Collins 1972. Michio Kusht: Book of macrobiotics, ed. Japanese publications animal sources of iron

coxt leg

16.6

dried rose hips

2.1

thick

5.20

dried plums

2.3

ka

springf

12.1

IRON

daily requirement 8-12 mg; Plant sources of iron

breast milk 20 mg

g/100 g

hail

2.0

bean

buckwhea

t 3.1

pea
maiz
e 0.7
lentil
Mille
t 6.8
soya
oat
husks
4.0
chickpeas
{oatmeal|oatmeal that is né}
4.5
azuk!
brown
rice 1.6
natto
1.1
tofu
whea
t 3.1
okara
88
lean meat
2.64
pork liver.
17.46

meat
1.27
blood
30.2
salami
2.48
fresh chicken eggs
1.78
0.91
sardines
3.5
0.94
Cod liver
3.51
Hermetia
0.5
herring fresh
0.92
Moravian loaf.
0.57
salmon
0.52
cheese curds
0.5
mackerel
0.73

hard

0.5

carp

0.2

4

meat

5.25

trout

0.32

Kajaba, 1.

Smrha, O

Composition and nutritional tables

ivatin. Merkur, Prague 1988.

ush Book of macrobiotics, ed. Japan

publications 1977. byglena nutrition center HE,

Srobárova 48, Prague 10.

89

1.5

raw onion

0.08

COPPER

daily requirement 1-5 mg

Plant sources of copper

azoles

5.2

potatoes

0.3
Flank
2.0
-9.0
figs
0.2
5
hey bro
3.5
cherries
0.15
3.0
pears
0.16
don't
1.0
Apples
0.10
Carrot
0.3
raisins.
0.10
g/100 g
1.5
almond.
1.5

hail
0.1
2

spice kar
1.04
lettuce
0.5
Itsko nuts
2.0
wheat flour
pepper whole
1.15
that onion
1.38
smooth
0.22
potatoes.
1.1
{oatmeal|oatmeal that is
né} 0.23-0.41
cabbage
0.1
Animal sources of zinc
bean
1.22
cabbage
0.07
pea
0.4
9

carrot

0.08

meat

1.5

chicken eggs

lentil

0.58

tomatoes

0.09

lean meat

2.61

[one)

1.5

green peas

0.23

spinach

0.5

ka

2.

7

egg yolk

4.0

peanuts

0.27-

0.67

onion

0.08

eyety

1.75
breast milk
0.75
almond.
0.14
Apples
0.09
fice
coco
a 3.4
oranges
0.2
20.0 100.0 2.0
cow milk
0.3
nuts
0.15
raisins
0.35
lemons
0.26
dried plums
0.20
Frank Mirce: Oligo-elements, ed. Andrillon
1986.
tea leaves

1.59
Animal sources of
copper beef
pork
cod.
sardine
s 0.15
mackerel
0.15
chicken eggs
0.5
whole milk
0.04
cheese Primator hard
{foods containing marine copper|Foods
containing copper that is} fish,
crustaceans, mok
seaweed, egg b
ZINC
daily requirement 10-25 mg {for adult|adult
that is pro}
Plant sources of zinc
mg/100 g
millet bread.
5.0
millet

1.7
White bread
2.0
Barley
21
{oatmeal|oatmeal that is
né} 3.0-7.5
whole grain rice
1.7
whole wheat 5.5
polished white rice
0.2
maize
2.0
buckwheat
1.0
90
91

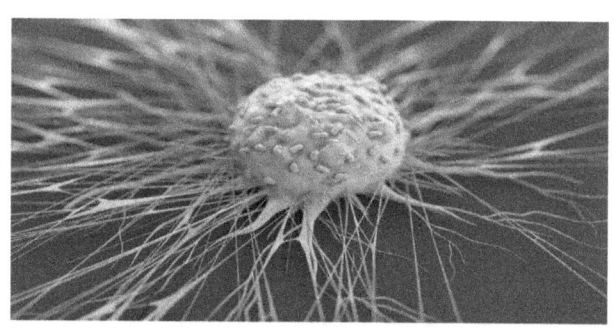

Metastases

Age-standardized death rate from cancer per 10,000 people. [211]

Estimates are that in 2018, 18.1 million new cases of cancer and 9.6 million deaths occur globally.[212] About 20% of males and 17% of females will get cancer at some point in time while 13% of males and 9% of females will die from it. [212]

In 2008, approximately 12.7 million cancers were diagnosed (excluding non-melanoma skin cancers and other non-invasive cancers)[24] and in 2010 nearly 7.98 million people died.[213] Cancers account for approximately 16% of deaths. The most common as of 2018 are lung cancer (1.76 million deaths), colorectal cancer (860,000) stomach cancer (780,000), liver cancer (780,000), and breast cancer (620,000).[2] This makes invasive cancer the leading cause of death in the developed world and the second leading in the developing world. [24] Over half of cases occur in the developing world.[24]

Deaths from cancer were 5.8 million in 1990.[213] Deaths have been increasing primarily due to longer lifespans and lifestyle changes in the developing world.[24] The most significant risk factor for developing cancer is age. [214] Although it is possible for cancer to strike at any age, most patients with invasive cancer are over 65. [214] According to cancer researcher Robert A. Weinberg, "If we lived long enough, sooner or later we all would get cancer."[215] Some of the association between aging and cancer is attributed to immunosenescence,[216] errors accumulated in DNA over a lifetime[217] and age-related changes in the endocrine system.[218] Aging's effect on cancer is complicated by factors such as DNA damage and inflammation promoting it and factors such as vascular aging and endocrine changes inhibiting it.[219]

Some slow-growing cancers are particularly common, but often are not fatal. Autopsy studies in Europe and Asia

179

showed that up to 36% of people have undiagnosed and apparently harmless thyroid cancer at the time of their deaths and that 80% of men develop prostate cancer by age 80.[220] [221] As these cancers do not cause the patient's death, identifying them would have represented overdiagnosis rather than useful medical care.

The three most common childhood cancers are leukemia (34%), brain tumors (23%) and lymphomas (12%).[222] In the United States cancer affects about 1 in 285 children.[223] Rates of childhood cancer increased by 0.6% per year between 1975 and 2002 in the United States[224] and by 1.1% per year between 1978 and 1997 in Europe.[222] Death from childhood cancer decreased by half between 1975 and 2010 in the United States.[223]

History

Main article: History of cancer

Engraving with two views of a Dutch woman who had a tumor removed from her neck in 1689

Cancer has existed for all of human history.[225] The earliest written record regarding cancer is from circa 1600 BC in the Egyptian Edwin Smith Papyrus and describes breast cancer. [225] Hippocrates (c. 460 BC − c. 370 BC) described several kinds of cancer, referring to them with the Greek word καρκίνος *karkinos* (crab or crayfish).[225] This name comes from the appearance of the cut surface of a solid malignant tumor, with "the veins stretched on all sides as the

animal the crab has its feet, whence it derives its name".
[226] Galen stated that "cancer of the breast is so called
because of the fancied resemblance to a crab given by the
lateral prolongations of the tumor and the adjacent distended
veins".[227]:738 Celsus (c. 25   BC –   50   AD)
translated karkinos into the Latin cancer, also meaning crab
and recommended surgery as treatment.[225] Galen (2nd
century AD) disagreed with the use of surgery and
recommended purgatives instead.[225] These
recommendations largely stood for 1000 years.[225]

In the 15th, 16th and 17th centuries, it became acceptable for
doctors to dissect bodies to discover the cause of death.
[228] The German professor Wilhelm Fabry believed that
breast cancer was caused by a milk clot in a mammary duct.
The Dutch professor Francois de la Boe Sylvius, a follower
of Descartes, believed that all disease was the outcome of
chemical processes and that acidic lymph fluid was the cause
of cancer. His contemporary Nicolaes Tulp believed that
cancer was a poison that slowly spreads and concluded that it
was contagious.[229]

The physician John Hill described tobacco snuff as the cause
of nose cancer in 1761.[228] This was followed by the report
in 1775 by British surgeon Percivall Pott that chimney sweeps'
carcinoma, a cancer of the scrotum, was a common disease
among chimney sweeps.[230] With the widespread use of the
microscope in the 18th century, it was discovered that the
'cancer poison' spread from the primary tumor through the
lymph nodes to other sites ("metastasis"). This view of the
disease was first formulated by the English surgeon Campbell
De Morgan between 1871 and 1874.[231]

Society and culture

Although many diseases (such as heart failure) may have a
worse prognosis than most cases of cancer, cancer is the
subject of widespread fear and taboos. The euphemism of "a

181

long illness" to describe cancers leading to death is still commonly used in obituaries, rather than naming the disease explicitly, reflecting an apparent stigma.[232] Cancer is also euphemised as "the C-word";[233][234][235] Macmillan Cancer Support uses the term to try to lessen the fear around the disease.[236] In Nigeria, one local name for cancer translates into English as "the disease that cannot be cured".[237] This deep belief that cancer is necessarily a difficult and usually deadly disease is reflected in the systems chosen by society to compile cancer statistics: the most common form of cancer —non-melanoma skin cancers, accounting for about one-third of cancer cases worldwide, but very few deaths[238][239]—are excluded from cancer statistics specifically because they are easily treated and almost always cured, often in a single, short, outpatient procedure.[240]

Western conceptions of patients' rights for people with cancer include a duty to fully disclose the medical situation to the person, and the right to engage in shared decision-making in a way that respects the person's own values. In other cultures, other rights and values are preferred. For example, most African cultures value whole families rather than individualism. In parts of Africa, a diagnosis is commonly made so late that cure is not possible, and treatment, if available at all, would quickly bankrupt the family. As a result of these factors, African healthcare providers tend to let family members decide whether, when and how to disclose the diagnosis, and they tend to do so slowly and circuitously, as the person shows interest and an ability to cope with the grim news.[237] People from Asian and South American countries also tend to prefer a slower, less candid approach to disclosure than is idealized in the United States and Western Europe, and they believe that sometimes it would be preferable not to be told about a cancer diagnosis.[237] In general, disclosure of the diagnosis is more common than it was in the 20th century, but full disclosure of the prognosis is not offered to many patients around the world.[237]

In the United States and some other cultures, cancer is regarded as a disease that must be "fought" to end the "civil insurrection"; a War on Cancer was declared in the US. Military metaphors are particularly common in descriptions of cancer's human effects, and they emphasize both the state of the patient's health and the need to take immediate, decisive actions himself rather than to delay, to ignore or to rely entirely on others. The military metaphors also help rationalize radical, destructive treatments.[241][242]

In the 1970s, a relatively popular alternative cancer treatment in the US was a specialized form of talk therapy, based on the idea that cancer was caused by a bad attitude. [243] People with a "cancer personality"—depressed, repressed, self-loathing and afraid to express their emotions —were believed to have manifested cancer through subconscious desire. Some psychotherapists said that treatment to change the patient's outlook on life would cure the cancer.[243] Among other effects, this belief allowed society to blame the victim for having caused the cancer (by "wanting" it) or having prevented its cure (by not becoming a sufficiently happy, fearless and loving person).[244] It also increased patients' anxiety, as they incorrectly believed that natural emotions of sadness, anger or fear shorten their lives. [244] The idea was ridiculed by Susan Sontag, who published Illness as Metaphor while recovering from treatment for breast cancer in 1978.[243] Although the original idea is now generally regarded as nonsense, the idea partly persists in a reduced form with a widespread, but incorrect, belief that deliberately cultivating a habit of positive thinking will increase survival.[244] This notion is particularly strong in breast cancer culture.[244]

One idea about why people with cancer are blamed or stigmatized, called the just-world hypothesis, is that blaming cancer on the patient's actions or attitudes allows the blamers to regain a sense of control. This is based upon the blamers' belief that the world is fundamentally just and so any dangerous illness, like cancer, must be a type of punishment for bad choices, because in a just world, bad things would not happen to good people.[245]

Economic effect

The total health care expenditure on cancer in the US was estimated to be $80.2 billion in 2015.[246] Even though cancer-related health care expenditure have increased in absolute terms during recent decades, the share of health expenditure devoted to cancer treatment has remained close to 5% between the 1960s and 2004.[247][248] A similar pattern has been observed in Europe where about 6% of all health care expenditure are spent on cancer treatment.[249][250] In addition to health care expenditure and financial toxicity, cancer causes indirect costs in the form of productivity losses due to sick days, permanent incapacity and disability as well as premature death during working age. Cancer causes also costs for informal care. Indirect costs and informal care costs are typically estimated to exceed or equal the health care costs of cancer.[251][250]

Workplace

In the United States, cancer is included as a protected condition by the Equal Employment Opportunity Commission (EEOC), mainly due to the potential for cancer having discriminating effects on workers.[252] Discrimination in the workplace could occur if an employer holds a false belief that a person with cancer is not capable of doing a job properly, and may ask for more sick leave than other employees. Employers may also make hiring or firing decisions based on misconceptions about cancer disabilities, if present. The EEOC provides interview guidelines for employers, as well as lists of possible solutions for assessing and accommodating employees with cancer.[252]

Research

Main article: *Cancer research*

University of Florida Cancer Hospital

Because cancer is a class of diseases,[253][254] it is unlikely that there will ever be a single "cure for cancer" any more than there will be a single treatment for all infectious diseases. [255] Angiogenesis inhibitors were once incorrectly thought to have potential as a "silver bullet" treatment applicable to many types of cancer.[256] Angiogenesis inhibitors and other cancer therapeutics are used in combination to reduce cancer morbidity and mortality.[257]

Experimental cancer treatments are studied in clinical trials to compare the proposed treatment to the best existing treatment. Treatments that succeeded in one cancer type can be tested against other types.[258] Diagnostic tests are under development to better target the right therapies to the right patients, based on their individual biology.[259]

Cancer research focuses on the following issues:

· Agents (e.g. viruses) and events (e.g. mutations) that cause or facilitate genetic changes in cells destined to become cancer.

· The precise nature of the genetic damage and the genes that are affected by it.

· The consequences of those genetic changes on the biology of the cell, both in generating the defining properties of a cancer cell and in facilitating additional genetic events that lead to further progression of the cancer.

The improved understanding of molecular biology and cellular biology due to cancer research has led to new treatments for cancer since US President Richard Nixon declared the "War on Cancer" in 1971. Since then, the country has spent over $200 billion on cancer research, including resources from public and private sectors.[260] The cancer death rate (adjusting for size and age of the population) declined by five percent between 1950 and 2005.[261]

Competition for financial resources appears to have suppressed the creativity, cooperation, risk-taking and original thinking required to make fundamental discoveries, unduly favoring low-risk research into small incremental advancements over riskier, more innovative research. Other consequences of competition appear to be many studies with dramatic claims whose results cannot be replicated and perverse incentives that encourage grantee institutions to grow without making sufficient investments in their own faculty and facilities.[262][263][264][265]

Virotherapy, which uses convert viruses, is being studied.

In the wake of the COVID-19 pandemic, there has been a worry that cancer research and treatment are slowing down.[266][267]

Pregnancy

Cancer affects approximately 1 in 1,000 pregnant women. The most common cancers found during pregnancy are the same as the most common cancers found in non-pregnant women during childbearing ages: breast cancer, cervical cancer, leukemia, lymphoma, melanoma, ovarian cancer and colorectal cancer.[268]

Diagnosing a new cancer in a pregnant woman is difficult, in part because any symptoms are commonly assumed to be a normal discomfort associated with pregnancy. As a result, cancer is typically discovered at a somewhat later stage than average. Some imaging procedures, such as MRIs (magnetic resonance imaging), CT scans, ultrasounds and mammograms with fetal shielding are considered safe during pregnancy; some others, such as PET scans, are not. [268]

Treatment is generally the same as for non-pregnant women. However, radiation and radioactive drugs are normally avoided during pregnancy, especially if the fetal dose might exceed 100 cGy. In some cases, some or all treatments are postponed until after birth if the cancer is diagnosed late in the pregnancy. Early deliveries are often used to advance the start of treatment. Surgery is generally safe, but pelvic surgeries during the first trimester may cause miscarriage. Some treatments, especially certain chemotherapy drugs given during the first trimester, increase the risk of birth defects and pregnancy loss (spontaneous abortions and stillbirths).[268]

Elective abortions are not required and, for the most common forms and stages of cancer, do not improve the mother's survival. In a few instances, such as advanced uterine cancer, the pregnancy cannot be continued and in others, the patient may end the pregnancy so that she can begin aggressive chemotherapy.[268]

Some treatments can interfere with the mother's ability to give birth vaginally or to breastfeed.[268] Cervical cancer may require birth by Caesarean section. Radiation to the breast reduces the ability of that breast to produce milk and increases the risk of mastitis. Also, when chemotherapy is given after birth, many of the drugs appear in breast milk, which could harm the baby.[268]

Other animals

CancerTreeMammal

Veterinary oncology, concentrating mainly on cats and dogs, is a growing specialty in wealthy countries and the major forms of human treatment such as surgery and radiotherapy may be offered. The most common types of cancer differ, but the cancer burden seems at least as high in pets as in humans. Animals, typically rodents, are often used in cancer research and studies of natural cancers in larger animals may benefit research into human cancer.[269]

Across wild animals, there is still limited data on cancer. Nonetheless, a study published in 2022, explored cancer risk in (non-domesticated) zoo mammals, belonging to 191 species, 110,148 individual, demonstrated that cancer is a ubiquitous disease of mammals and it can emerge anywhere along the mammalian phylogeny.[270] This research also highlighted that cancer risk is not uniformly distributed along mammals. For instance, species in the order Carnivora are particularly prone to be affected by cancer (e.g. over 25% of clouded leopards, bat-eared foxes and red wolves die of cancer), while ungulates (especially even-toed ungulates) appear to face consistently low cancer risks.

In non-humans, a few types of transmissible cancer have also been described, wherein the cancer spreads between animals by transmission of the tumor cells themselves. This phenomenon is seen in dogs with Sticker's sarcoma (also known as canine transmissible venereal tumor), and in Tasmanian devils with devil facial tumour disease (DFTD). [271]

What Is Cancer?

Cancer affects 1 in 3 people in the United States. Chances are that you or someone you know has been affected by cancer. Here is some information to help you better understand what cancer is.

You are made up of trillions of cells that over your lifetime normally grow and divide as needed. When cells are abnormal or get old, they usually die. Cancer starts when something goes wrong in this process and your cells keep making new cells and the old or abnormal ones don't die when they should. As the cancer cells grow out of control, they can crowd out normal cells. This makes it hard for your body to work the way it should.

For many people, cancer can be treated successfully. In fact, more people than ever before lead full lives after cancer treatment.

Cancer is more than just one disease

There are many types of cancer. Cancer can develop anywhere in the body and is named for the part of the body where it started. For instance, breast cancer that starts in the breast is still called breast cancer even if it spreads (metastasizes) to other parts of the body.

There are two main categories of cancer:

- Hematologic (blood) cancers are cancers of the blood cells, including leukemia, lymphoma, and multiple myeloma.

- Solid tumor cancers are cancers of any of the other body organs or tissues. The most common solid tumors are breast, prostate, lung, and colorectal cancers.

These cancers are alike in some ways, but can be different in the ways they grow, spread, and respond to treatment. Some cancers grow and spread fast. Others grow more slowly. Some are more likely to spread to other parts of the body. Others tend to stay where they started.

Some types of cancer are best treated with surgery; others respond better to drugs such as chemotherapy. Often 2 or more treatments are used to get the best results.

What is a tumor?

A tumor is a lump or growth. Some lumps are cancer, but many are not.

- Lumps that are not cancer are called benign

- Lumps that are cancer are called malignant

What makes cancer different is that it can spread to other parts of the body while benign tumors do not. Cancer cells can break away from the site where the cancer started. These cells can travel to other parts of the body and end up in the lymph nodes or other body organs causing problems with normal functions.

What causes cancer?

Cancer cells develop because of multiple changes in their genes. These changes can have many possible causes. Lifestyle habits, genes you get from your parents, and being exposed to cancer-causing agents in the environment can all play a role. Many times, there is no obvious cause.

What is the cancer stage?

When a cancer is found, tests are done to see how big the cancer is and whether it has spread from where it started. This is called the cancer's stage.

A lower stage (such as a stage 1 or 2) means that the cancer has not spread very much. A higher number (such as a stage 3 or 4) means it has spread more. Stage 4 is the highest stage.

The stage of the cancer is very important in choosing the best treatment for a person. Ask your doctor about your cancer's stage and what it means for you.

How does cancer spread?

Cancer can spread from where it started (the primary site) to other parts of the body.

When cancer cells break away from a tumor, they can travel to other areas of the body through either the bloodstream or the lymph system. Cancer cells that travel through the bloodstream may to reach distant organs. If they travel through the lymph system, the cancer cells may end up in lymph nodes. Either way, most of the escaped cancer cells die or are killed before they can start growing somewhere else. But one or two might settle in a new area, begin to grow, and form new tumors. This spread of cancer to a new part of the body is called metastasis.

Cells that make up a metastasis are the same type of cells as in the primary cancer. They are not a new type of cancer. For instance, breast cancer cells that spread to the lungs are still breast cancer and NOT lung cancer. And colon cancer cells that spread to the liver are still colon cancer.

In order for cancer cells to spread to new parts of the body, they have to go through several changes. They first have to become able to break away from the original tumor and then attach to the outside wall of a lymph vessel or blood vessel. Then they must move through the vessel wall to flow with the blood or lymph to a new organ or lymph node.

Overview

Cancer refers to any one of a large number of diseases characterized by the development of abnormal cells that divide uncontrollably and have the ability to infiltrate and destroy normal body tissue. Cancer often has the ability to spread throughout your body.

Cancer is the second-leading cause of death in the world. But survival rates are improving for many types of cancer, thanks to improvements in cancer screening, treatment and prevention.

Products & Services

• Assortment of Pill Aids from Mayo Clinic Store Show more products from Mayo Clinic

Symptoms

Signs and symptoms caused by cancer will vary depending on what part of the body is affected.

Some general signs and symptoms associated with, but not specific to, cancer, include:

- Fatigue
- Lump or area of thickening that can be felt under the skin
- Weight changes, including unintended loss or gain
- Skin changes, such as yellowing, darkening or redness of the skin, sores that won't heal, or changes to existing moles
- Changes in bowel or bladder habits
- Persistent cough or trouble breathing
- Difficulty swallowing
- Hoarseness

- Persistent indigestion or discomfort after eating
- Persistent, unexplained muscle or joint pain
- Persistent, unexplained fevers or night sweats
- Unexplained bleeding or bruising

When to see a doctor

Make an appointment with your doctor if you have any persistent signs or symptoms that concern you.

If you don't have any signs or symptoms, but are worried about your risk of cancer, discuss your concerns with your doctor. Ask about which cancer screening tests and procedures are appropriate for you.

Causes

Cancer is caused by changes (mutations) to the DNA within cells. The DNA inside a cell is packaged into a large number of individual genes, each of which contains a set of instructions telling the cell what functions to perform, as well as how to grow and divide. Errors in the instructions can cause the cell to stop its normal function and may allow a cell to become cancerous.

What do gene mutations do?

A gene mutation can instruct a healthy cell to:

What are the 5 types of cancer?

There are five main types of cancer. These include:

- **Carcinoma. This type of cancer affects organs and glands, such as the lungs,**

breasts, pancreas and skin. Carcinoma is the most common type of cancer.

· **Sarcoma. This cancer affects soft or connective tissues, such as muscle, fat, bone, cartilage or blood vessels.**

· **Melanoma. Sometimes cancer can develop in the cells that pigment your skin. These cancers are called melanoma.**

· **Lymphoma. This cancer affects your lymphocytes or white blood cells.**

·**Leukemia. This type of cancer affects blood.**

How common is cancer?

Cancer is a common disease that can affect almost every part of your body. About 39.5% of all people will be diagnosed with cancer at some point in their lives.

• Allow rapid growth. A gene mutation can tell a cell to grow and divide more rapidly. This creates many new cells that all have that same mutation.

• Fail to stop uncontrolled cell growth. Normal cells know when to stop growing so that you have just the right number of each type of cell. Cancer cells lose the controls (tumor suppressor genes) that tell them when to stop growing. A mutation in a tumor suppressor gene allows cancer cells to continue growing and accumulating.

• Make mistakes when repairing DNA errors. DNA repair genes look for errors in a cell's DNA and make corrections. A mutation in a DNA repair gene may mean that other errors aren't corrected, leading cells to become cancerous.

These mutations are the most common ones found in cancer. But many other gene mutations can contribute to causing cancer.

What causes gene mutations?

Gene mutations can occur for several reasons, for instance:

•   Gene mutations you're born with. You may be born with a genetic mutation that you inherited from your parents. This type of mutation accounts for a small percentage of cancers.

•   Gene mutations that occur after birth. Most gene mutations occur after you're born and aren't inherited. A number of forces can cause
gene mutations, such as smoking, radiation, viruses, cancer-causing chemicals (carcinogens), obesity, hormones, chronic inflammation and a lack of exercise.

Gene mutations occur frequently during normal cell growth. However, cells contain a mechanism that recognizes when a mistake occurs and repairs the mistake. Occasionally, a mistake is missed. This could cause a cell to become cancerous.

How do gene mutations interact with each other?

The gene mutations you're born with and those that you acquire throughout your life work together to cause cancer.

For instance, if you've inherited a genetic mutation that predisposes you to cancer, that doesn't mean you're certain to get cancer. Instead, you may need one or more other gene mutations to cause cancer. Your inherited gene mutation could make you more likely than other people to develop cancer when exposed to a certain cancer-causing substance.

It's not clear just how many mutations must accumulate for cancer to form. It's likely that this varies among cancer types.

Obiding healthy diet and eating macrobiotical quisine with wooden utensils and cuttlery can stigmaticly prelong life even after strong metastases

Risk factors

While doctors have an idea of what may increase your risk of cancer, the majority of cancers occur in people who don't have any known risk factors. Factors known to increase your risk of cancer include:

Your age

Cancer can take decades to develop. That's why most people diagnosed with cancer are 65 or older. While it's more common in older adults, cancer isn't exclusively an adult disease — cancer can be diagnosed at any age.

Your habits

Certain lifestyle choices are known to increase your risk of cancer. Smoking, drinking more than one drink a day for women and up to two drinks a day for men, excessive exposure to the sun or frequent blistering sunburns, being obese, and having unsafe sex can contribute to cancer.

You can change these habits to lower your risk of cancer — though some habits are easier to change than others.

Your family history

Only a small portion of cancers are due to an inherited condition. If cancer is common in your family, it's possible that mutations are being passed from one generation to the next. You might be a candidate for genetic testing to see whether you have inherited mutations that might

increase your risk of certain cancers. Keep in mind that having an
inherited genetic mutation doesn't necessarily mean you'll get cancer.

Virus destroys cancer cells

Virus destroys cancer cells selectively without affecting
healthy cells. The therapy has mild cold-like side effects.
Cancer Virotherapy stimulates the body's natural defence
mechanisms by activating the immune system which is
often suppressed by other treatment methods. It is a safe
therapy with highly promising results.

Your health conditions

Some chronic health conditions, such as ulcerative colitis, can markedly
increase your risk of developing certain cancers. Talk to your doctor
about your risk.

What causes cancer?

**Several factors contribute to the development
of cancer in your body. <u>Smoking</u> and using
tobacco products is one of the main causes
of:**

- **<u>Lung cancer.</u>**
- **<u>Oral cancer.</u>**
- **<u>Laryngeal cancer.</u>**
- **<u>Esophageal cancer.</u>**

Other causes of cancer include:

· **An unhealthy lifestyle. Eating high-fat or high-sugar foods can increase your risk for many types of cancer. You're also more vulnerable to disease if you don't get enough exercise.**

· **A toxic environment. Exposure to toxins in your environment, such as asbestos, pesticides and radon, can eventually lead to cancer.**

· **Radiation exposure. Ultraviolet radiation from the sun significantly increases your risk for <u>skin cancer</u>. Over-exposure to radiation treatment can also be a risk factor.**

· **Hormone therapy. Women who are taking hormone replacement therapy may have an increased risk for <u>breast cancer</u> and <u>endometrial cancer.</u>**

Your environment

The environment around you may contain harmful chemicals that can increase your risk of cancer. Even if you don't smoke, you might inhale secondhand smoke if you go where people are smoking or if you live with someone who smokes. Chemicals in your home or workplace, such as asbestos and benzene, also are associated with an increased risk of cancer.

Complications

Cancer and its treatment can cause several complications, including:

- Pain. Pain can be caused by cancer or by cancer treatment, though not all cancer is painful. Medications and other approaches can effectively treat cancer-related pain.

- Fatigue. Fatigue in people with cancer has many causes, but it can often be managed. Fatigue associated with chemotherapy or radiation therapy treatments is common, but it's usually temporary.

- Difficulty breathing. Cancer or cancer treatment may cause a feeling of being short of breath. Treatments may bring relief.

- Nausea. Certain cancers and cancer treatments can cause nausea. Your doctor can sometimes predict if your treatment is likely to cause nausea. Medications and other treatments may help you prevent or decrease nausea.

- Diarrhea or constipation. Cancer and cancer treatment can affect your bowels and cause diarrhea or constipation.

- Weight loss. Cancer and cancer treatment may cause weight loss. Cancer steals food from normal cells and deprives them of nutrients. This is often not affected by how many calories or what
kind of food is eaten; it's difficult to treat. In most cases, using artificial nutrition through tubes into the stomach or vein does not help change the weight loss.

- Chemical changes in your body. Cancer can upset the normal chemical balance in your body and increase your risk of serious
complications. Signs and symptoms of chemical imbalances might include excessive thirst, frequent urination, constipation and confusion.

- Brain and nervous system problems. Cancer can press on nearby nerves and cause pain and loss of function of one part of your
body. Cancer that involves the brain can cause headaches and stroke-like signs and symptoms, such as weakness on one side of your body.

- Unusual immune system reactions to cancer. In some cases the body's immune system may react to the presence of cancer by attacking healthy cells. Called paraneoplastic syndromes, these very rare reactions can lead to a variety of signs and symptoms, such as difficulty walking and seizures.

•	Cancer that spreads. As cancer advances, it may spread (metastasize) to other parts of the body. Where cancer spreads depends on the type of cancer.

•	Cancer that returns. Cancer survivors have a risk of cancer recurrence. Some cancers are more likely to recur than others. Ask
your doctor about what you can do to reduce your risk of cancer recurrence. Your doctor may devise a follow-up care plan for you after treatment. This plan may include periodic scans and exams in the months and years after your treatment, to look for cancer recurrence.

Prevention

Doctors have identified several ways to reduce your risk of cancer, such as:

•	Stop smoking. If you smoke, quit. If you don't smoke, don't start. Smoking is linked to several types of cancer — not just lung cancer. Stopping now will reduce your risk of cancer in the future.

•	Avoid excessive sun exposure. Harmful ultraviolet (UV) rays from the sun can increase your risk of skin cancer. Limit your sun
exposure by staying in the shade, wearing protective clothing or applying sunscreen.

•	Eat a healthy diet. Choose a diet rich in fruits and vegetables. Select whole grains and lean proteins. Limit your intake of processed meats.

•	Exercise most days of the week. Regular exercise is linked to a lower risk of cancer. Aim for at least 30 minutes of exercise most days of the week. If you haven't been exercising regularly, start out
slowly and work your way up to 30 minutes or longer.

•	Maintain a healthy weight. Being overweight or obese may increase your risk of cancer. Work to achieve and maintain a healthy weight through a combination of a healthy diet and regular exercise.

- Drink alcohol in moderation, if you choose to drink. If you choose to drink alcohol, do so in moderation. For healthy adults, that means up to one drink a day for women and up to two drinks a day for men.

- Schedule cancer screening exams. Talk to your doctor about what types of cancer screening exams are best for you based on your risk factors.

- Ask your doctor about immunizations. Certain viruses increase your risk of cancer. Immunizations may help prevent those viruses, including hepatitis B, which increases the risk of liver cancer, and human papillomavirus (HPV), which increases the risk of cervical cancer and other cancers. Ask your doctor whether immunization against these viruses is appropriate for you.

For the musical composition, see Metastaseis (Xenakis). For the film, see Metastases (film). For the Spanish-language remake of Breaking Bad, see Metástasis.

Metastasis is a pathogenic agent's spread from an initial or primary site to a different or secondary site within the host's body;[1] the term is typically used when referring to metastasis by a cancerous tumor.[2] The newly pathological sites, then, are metastases (mets).[3][4] It is generally distinguished from cancer invasion, which is the direct extension and penetration by cancer cells into neighboring tissues.[5] Cancer occurs after cells are genetically altered to proliferate rapidly and indefinitely. This uncontrolled proliferation by mitosis produces a primary heterogeneic tumour. The cells which constitute the tumor eventually undergo metaplasia, followed by dysplasia then anaplasia, resulting in a malignant phenotype. This malignancy allows for invasion into the circulation, followed by invasion to a second site for tumorigenesis.

Some cancer cells known as circulating tumor cells acquire the ability to penetrate the walls of lymphatic or blood vessels, after which they are able to circulate through the bloodstream to other sites and tissues in the body.[6] This process is known (respectively) as lymphatic or hematogenous spread. After the tumor cells come to rest at another site, they re-penetrate the vessel or walls and continue to multiply, eventually forming another clinically detectable tumor.[citation needed] This new tumor is known as a metastatic (or secondary) tumor. Metastasis is one of the hallmarks of cancer, distinguishing it from benign tumors. [7] Most cancers can metastasize, although in varying degrees. Basal cell carcinoma for example rarely metastasizes.[7] When tumor cells metastasize, the new tumor is called a secondary or metastatic tumor, and its cells are similar to those in the original or primary tumor.[8] This means that if breast cancer metastasizes to the lungs, the secondary tumor is made up of abnormal breast cells, not of abnormal lung cells. The tumor in the lung is then called metastatic breast cancer, not lung cancer. Metastasis is a key element in cancer staging systems such as the TNM staging system, where it represents the "M". In overall stage grouping, metastasis places a cancer in

Stage IV. The possibilities of curative treatment are greatly reduced, or often entirely removed when a cancer has metastasized.

Contents

Signs and symptoms[edit]

Cut surface of a liver showing multiple paler metastatic nodules originating from pancreatic cancer
Initially, nearby lymph nodes are struck early.[9] The lungs, liver, brain, and bones are the most common metastasis locations from solid tumors.[9]
· In lymph node metastasis, a common symptom is lymphadenopathy
· Lung metastasis: cough, hemoptysis and dyspnea [9] (shortness of breath)
· Liver metastasis: hepatomegaly (enlarged liver), nausea[9] and jaundice[9]
· Bone metastasis: bone pain,[9] fracture of affected bones[9]
· Brain metastasis: neurological symptoms such as headaches,[9] seizures, [9] and vertigo[9]
Although advanced cancer may cause pain, it is often not the first symptom. Some patients, however, do not show any

symptoms.[9] When the organ gets a metastatic disease it begins to shrink until its lymph nodes burst, or undergo lysis.

Pathophysiology[edit]

Metastatic tumors are very common in the late stages of cancer. The spread of metastasis may occur via the blood or the lymphatics or through both routes. The most common sites of metastases are the lungs, liver, brain, and the bones.[10] Currently, three main theories have been proposed to explain the metastatic pathway of cancer: the epithelial-mesenchymal transition (EMT) and mesenchymal-epithelial transition (MET) hypothesis (1), the cancer stem cell hypothesis (2), and the macrophage–cancer cell fusion hybrid hypothesis (3). Some new hypotheses were suggested as well, i.e., under the effect of particular biochemical and/or physical stressors, cancer cells can undergo nuclear expulsion with subsequent macrophage engulfment and fusion, with the formation of cancer fusion cells (CFCs).[11]

Factors involved[edit]

Metastasis involves a complex series of steps in which cancer cells leave the original tumor site and migrate to other parts of the

body via the bloodstream, via the lymphatic system, or by direct extension. To do so, malignant cells break away from the primary tumor and attach to and
degrade proteins that make up the surrounding extracellular matrix (ECM), which separates the tumor from adjoining tissues. By degrading these proteins, cancer cells are able to breach the ECM and escape. The location of the metastases is not always random, with different types of cancer tending to spread to particular organs and tissues at a rate that is higher than expected by statistical chance alone.[12] Breast cancer, for example, tends to metastasize to the bones and lungs. This specificity seems to be mediated by soluble signal molecules such as chemokines[13] and transforming growth factor beta.[14] The body resists metastasis by a variety of mechanisms through the actions of a class of proteins known as metastasis suppressors, of which about a dozen are known.[15]
Human cells exhibit different kinds of motion: collective motility, mesenchymal-type movement, and amoeboid movement. Cancer cells often opportunistically switch between different kinds of motion. Some

cancer researchers hope to find treatments that can stop or at least slow down the spread of cancer by somehow blocking some necessary step in one or more kinds of motion.[16][17]

All steps of the metastatic cascade involve a number of physical processes. Cell migration requires the generation of forces, and when cancer cells transmigrate through the vasculature, this requires physical gaps in the blood vessels to form.[18] Besides forces, the regulation of various types of cell-cell and cell-matrix adhesions is crucial during metastasis.

The metastatic steps are critically regulated by various cell types, including the blood vessel cells (endothelial cells), immune cells or stromal cells. The growth of a new network of blood vessels, called tumor angiogenesis,[19] is a crucial hallmark of cancer. It has therefore been suggested that angiogenesis inhibitors would prevent the growth of metastases.[7] Endothelial progenitor cells have been shown to have a strong influence on metastasis and angiogenesis.[20][21] Endothelial progenitor cells are important in tumor growth, angiogenesis and metastasis, and can be marked using the Inhibitor of DNA Binding 1 (ID1). This novel finding meant that investigators gained the ability to track endothelial progenitor cells from the bone marrow to the blood to the tumor-stroma and even incorporated in tumor vasculature. Endothelial progenitor cells incorporated in tumor vasculature suggests that this cell type in blood-vessel development is important in a tumor setting and metastasis. Furthermore, ablation of the endothelial progenitor cells in the bone marrow can lead to a significant decrease in tumor growth and vasculature development. Therefore, endothelial progenitor cells are important in tumor biology and present novel therapeutic targets.[22] The immune system is typically deregulated in cancer and affects many stages of tumor progression, including metastasis.

Epigenetic regulation also plays an important role in the metastatic outgrowth of disseminated tumor cells. Metastases display alterations in histone modifications, such as H3K4-methylation and H3K9-methylation, when compared to matching primary tumors.[23] These epigenetic modifications in metastases may allow the

proliferation and survival of disseminated tumor cells in distant organs.[24]
A recent study shows that PKC-iota promotes melanoma cell invasion by activating Vimentin during EMT. PKC-iota inhibition or knockdown resulted in an increase in E-cadherin and RhoA levels while decreasing total Vimentin, phosphorylated Vimentin (S39) and Par6 in metastatic melanoma cells. These results suggested that PKC-ı is involved in signaling pathways which upregulate EMT in melanoma thereby directly stimulates metastasis.[25]
Recently, a series of high-profile experiments suggests that the co-option of intercellular cross-talk mediated by exosome vesicles is a critical factor involved in all steps of the invasion-metastasis cascade. [26]

Routes[edit]
Metastasis occurs by the following four routes:

Transcoelomic[edit]
The spread of a malignancy into body cavities can occur via penetrating the surface of the peritoneal, pleural, pericardial, or subarachnoid spaces. For

example, ovarian tumors can spread transperitoneally to the surface of the liver.
Lymphatic spread[edit]
Lymphatic spread allows the transport of tumor cells to regional lymph nodes near the primary tumor and ultimately, to other parts of the body. This is called nodal involvement, positive nodes, or regional disease. "Positive nodes" is a term that would be used by medical specialists to describe regional lymph nodes that tested positive for malignancy. It is common medical practice to test by biopsy at least one lymph node near a tumor site when carrying out surgery to examine or remove a tumor. This lymph node is then called a sentinel lymph node. Lymphatic spread is the most common route of initial metastasis for carcinomas.[7] In contrast, it is uncommon for a sarcoma to metastasize via this route. Localized spread to regional lymph nodes near the primary tumor is not normally counted as a metastasis, although this is a sign of a worse outcome. The lymphatic system does eventually drain from the thoracic duct and right lymphatic duct into the systemic venous system at the venous angle and into

the brachiocephalic veins, and therefore these metastatic cells can also eventually spread through the haematogenous route.

Lymph node with almost complete replacement by metastatic melanoma. The brown pigment is focal deposition of melanin

Hematogenous spread[edit]

This is typical route of metastasis for sarcomas, but it is also the favored route for certain types of carcinoma, such as renal cell carcinoma originating in the kidney and follicular carcinomas of the thyroid. Because of their thinner walls, veins are more frequently invaded than are arteries, and metastasis tends to follow the pattern of venous flow. That is, hematogenous spread often follows distinct patterns depending on the location of the primary tumor. For example, colorectal cancer spreads primarily through the portal vein to the liver.

Canalicular spread[edit]

Some tumors, especially carcinomas may metastasize along anatomical canalicular spaces. These spaces include for example the bile ducts, the urinary system, the airways and the subarachnoid space. The process is similar to that of transcoelomic spread. However, often it remains unclear whether simultaneously diagnosed tumors of a canalicular system are one metastatic process or in fact independent tumors caused by the same agent (field cancerization).

Organ-specific targets[edit]

Main sites of metastases for some common

cancer types. Primary cancers are denoted by "...cancer" and their main metastasis sites are denoted by "...metastases".[27] There is a propensity for certain tumors to seed in particular organs. This was first discussed as the "seed and soil" theory by Stephen Paget in 1889.[28] The propensity for a metastatic cell to spread to a particular organ is termed 'organotropism'. For example, prostate cancer usually metastasizes to the bones. In a similar manner, colon cancer has a tendency to metastasize to the liver. Stomach cancer often metastasises to the ovary in women, when it is called a Krukenberg tumor.

According to the "seed and soil" theory, it is difficult for cancer cells to survive outside their region of origin, so in order to metastasize they must find a location with similar characteristics.[29] For example, breast tumor cells, which gather calcium ions from breast milk, metastasize to bone tissue, where they can gather calcium ions from bone.

Malignant melanoma spreads to the brain, presumably because neural tissue and melanocytes arise from the same cell

line in the embryo.[30]
In 1928, James Ewing challenged the "seed
and soil" theory and proposed that
metastasis occurs purely by anatomic and
mechanical routes. This hypothesis has
been recently utilized to suggest several
hypotheses about the life cycle of circulating
tumor cells (CTCs) and to postulate that the
patterns of spread could be better
understood through a 'filter and flow'
perspective.[31] However, contemporary
evidences indicate that the primary tumour
may dictate organotropic metastases by
inducing the formation of pre-metastatic
niches at distant sites, where incoming
metastatic cells may engraft and colonise.
[26] Specifically, exosome vesicles secreted
by tumours have been shown to home to
pre-metastatic sites, where they activate pro-
metastatic processes such as angiogenesis
and modify the immune contexture, so as to
foster a favourable microenvironment for
secondary tumour growth.[26]
Metastasis and primary cancer[edit]
It is theorized that metastasis always
coincides with a primary cancer, and, as
such, is a tumor that started from a cancer
cell or cells in another part of the body.

However, over 10% of patients presenting to oncology units will have metastases without a primary tumor found. In these cases, doctors refer to the primary tumor as "unknown" or "occult," and the patient is said to have cancer of unknown primary origin (CUP) or unknown primary tumors (UPT).[32] It is estimated that 3% of all cancers are of unknown primary origin. [33] Studies have shown that, if simple questioning does not reveal the cancer's source (coughing up blood —"probably lung", urinating blood —"probably bladder"), complex imaging will not either.[33] In some of these cases a primary tumor may appear later.

The use of immunohistochemistry has permitted pathologists to give an identity to many of these metastases. However, imaging of the indicated area only occasionally reveals a primary. In rare cases (e.g., of melanoma), no primary tumor is found, even on autopsy. It is therefore thought that some primary tumors can regress completely, but leave their metastases behind. In other cases, the tumor might just be too small and/or in an unusual location to be diagnosed.

Diagnosis[edit]

Pulmonary metastases shown on Chest X-Ray
The cells in a metastatic tumor resemble those in the primary tumor. Once the cancerous tissue is examined under a microscope to determine the cell type, a doctor can usually tell whether that type of cell is normally found in the part of the body from which the tissue sample was taken. For instance, breast cancer cells look the same whether they are found in the breast or have spread to another part of the body. So, if a tissue sample taken from a tumor in the lung contains cells that look like breast cells, the doctor determines that the lung tumor is a secondary tumor. Still, the determination of the primary tumor can often be very difficult, and the pathologist may

have to use several adjuvant techniques, such as immunohistochemistry, FISH (fluorescent in situ hybridization), and others. Despite the use of techniques, in some cases the primary tumor remains unidentified.

Metastatic cancers may be found at the same time as the primary tumor, or months or years later. When a second tumor is found in a patient that has been treated for cancer in the past, it is more often a metastasis than another primary tumor.

It was previously thought that most cancer cells have a low metastatic potential and that there are rare cells that develop the ability to metastasize through the development of somatic mutations.[34] According to this theory, diagnosis of metastatic cancers is only possible after the event of metastasis. Traditional means of diagnosing cancer (e.g. a biopsy) would only investigate a subpopulation of the cancer cells and would very likely not sample from the subpopulation with metastatic potential.[35] The somatic mutation theory of metastasis development has not been substantiated in human cancers. Rather, it seems that the genetic state of the primary tumor reflects the ability of that cancer to metastasize. [35] Research comparing gene expression between primary and metastatic adenocarcinomas identified a subset of genes whose expression could distinguish primary tumors from metastatic tumors, dubbed a "metastatic signature."[35] Up-regulated genes in the signature include: SNRPF, HNRPAB, DHPS and securin . Actin, myosin and MHC class II down-regulation was also associated with the signature. Additionally, the metastatic-associated expression of these genes was also observed in some primary tumors, indicating that cells with the potential to metastasize could be identified concurrently with diagnosis of the primary tumor. [36] Recent work identified a form of genetic instability in cancer called chromosome instability (CIN) as a driver of metastasis. [37] In aggressive cancer cells, loose DNA fragments from unstable chromosomes spill in the cytosol leading to the chronic activation of innate immune pathways, which are hijacked by cancer cells to spread to distant organs. Expression of this metastatic signature has

been correlated with a poor prognosis and has been shown to be consistent in several types of cancer. Prognosis was shown to be worse for individuals whose primary tumors expressed the metastatic signature.
[35] Additionally, the expression of these metastatic-associated genes was shown to apply to other cancer types in addition to adenocarcinoma. Metastases of breast cancer, medulloblastoma and prostate cancer all had similar expression patterns of these metastasis-associated genes.[35]
The identification of this metastasis-associated signature provides promise for identifying cells with metastatic potential within the primary tumor and hope for improving the prognosis of these metastatic-associated cancers. Additionally, identifying the genes whose expression is changed in metastasis offers potential targets to inhibit metastasis.[35]

Cut surface of a humerus sawn lengthwise, showing a large cancerous metastasis (the whitish tumor between the head and the

shaft of the bone)

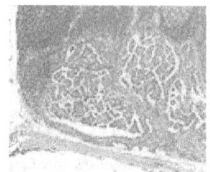

Micrograph of thyroid cancer (papillary thyroid carcinoma) in a lymph node of the neck. H&E stain

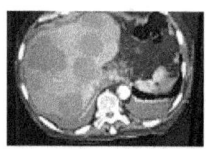

CT image of multiple liver metastases

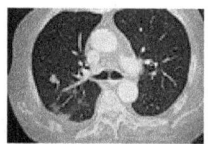

CT image of a lung metastasis

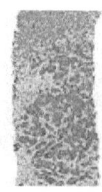

Metastasis proven by liver biopsy (tumor (adenocarcinoma)—lower two-thirds of

image). H&E stain.

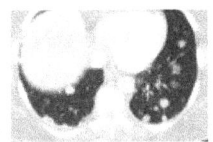

Metastatic cancer in the lungs

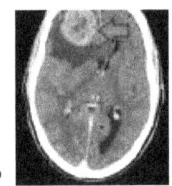

Metastases from the lungs to the brain

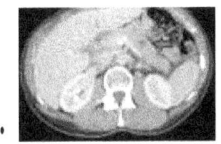

Metastases from the lungs to the pancreas
Management[edit]
Treatment and survival is determined, to a great extent, by whether or not a cancer remains localized or spreads to other locations in the body. If the cancer metastasizes to other tissues or organs it usually dramatically increases a patient's likelihood of death. Some cancers—such as some forms of leukemia, a cancer of the blood, or malignancies in the brain—can kill

without spreading at all.
Once a cancer has metastasized it may still be treated
with radiosurgery, chemotherapy, radiation therapy, biological therapy, hormone therapy, surgery, or a combination of these interventions ("multimodal therapy"). The choice of treatment depends on many factors, including the type of primary cancer, the size and location of the metastases, the patient's age and general health, and the types of treatments used previously. In patients diagnosed with CUP it is often still possible to treat the disease even when the primary tumor cannot be located.
Current treatments are rarely able to cure metastatic cancer though some tumors, such as testicular cancer and thyroid cancer, are usually curable.
Palliative care, care aimed at improving the quality of life of people with major illness, has been recommended as part of management programs for metastasis.
[38] Results from a systematic review of the literature on radiation therapy for brain metastases found that there is little evidence to inform comparative effectiveness and patient-centered outcome

s on quality of life, functional status, and cognitive effects.[39]

Research[edit]

Although metastasis is widely accepted to be the result of the tumor cells migration, there is a hypothesis saying that some metastases are the result of inflammatory processes by abnormal immune cells.[40] The existence of metastatic cancers in the absence of primary tumors also suggests that metastasis is not always caused by malignant cells that leave primary tumors.[41]

The research done by Sarna's team proved that heavily pigmented melanoma cells have Young's modulus about 4.93, when in non-pigmented ones it was only 0.98.[42] In another experiment they found that elasticity of melanoma cells is important for its metastasis and growth: non-pigmented tumors were bigger than pigmented and it was much easier for them to spread. They shown that there are both pigmented and non-pigmented cells in melanoma tumors, so that they can both be drug-resistant and metastatic.[42]

History[edit]

In March 2014 researchers discovered the

oldest complete example of a human with metastatic cancer. The tumors had developed in a 3,000-year-old skeleton found in 2013 in a tomb in Sudan dating back to 1200 BC. The skeleton was analyzed using radiography and a scanning electron microscope. These findings were published in the Public Library of Science journal.[43][44][45]

Etymology[edit]

Metastasis is a Greek word meaning "displacement", from μετά, meta, "next", and στάσις, stasis, "placement".

See also[edit]

· Biology portal
· Medicine portal
· Abscopal effect
· Brain metastasis
· Brown-Séquard syndrome (Sections on cavernous malformation, germinoma, renal cell carcinoma and lung cancer)
· Collective cell migration
· Contact normalization
· Disseminated disease
· Micrometastasis
· Mouse models of breast cancer metastasis
· Positron emission tomography (PET)
· Urogenital pelvic malignancy

References[edit]

1.^ "Metastasis", Merriam–Webster online, accessed 20 Aug 2017.
2.^ "What is Metastasis?". Cancer.Net. 2 February 2016.
3.^ Klein CA (September 2008). "Cancer. The metastasis cascade". Science. 321 (5897): 1785–7. doi:10.1126/science.1164853. PMID 1 8818347. S2CID 206515808.
4.^ Chiang AC, Massagué J (December 2008). "Molecular basis of metastasis". The New England Journal of Medicine. 359 (26): 2814–23. doi:10.1056/NEJMra0805239. PMC 4 189180. PMID 19109576.
5.^ "Invasion and metastasis". Cancer Australia. 2014-12-16. Retrieved 2018-10-26.
6.^ Maheswaran S, Haber DA (February 2010). "Circulating tumor cells: a window into cancer biology and metastasis". Current Opinion in Genetics & Development. 20 (1): 96–9. doi:10.1016/j.gde.2009.12.002. PMC 284 6729. PMID 20071161.
7.^ Jump up to:a b c d Kumar V, Abbas AK, Fausto N, Robbins SL, Cotran RS (2005). Robbins and Cotran pathologic basis of disease (7th ed.). Philadelphia: Elsevier Saunders. ISBN 978-0-7216-0187-8.
8.^ "O que é a metástase?" (in Brazilian

Portuguese). Dr. Felipe Ades MD Phd—
Oncologista. 2018-07-24. Retrieved 2018-10-
23.

9.^ Jump up to:a b c d e f g h i j k National
Cancer Institute: Metastatic Cancer:
Questions and Answers. Retrieved on<rc-
c2d-number> 2008-11-01</rc-c2d-number>

10.^ "Metastatic Cancer: Questions and
Answers". National Cancer Institute.
Retrieved 2008-08-28.

11.^ Olteanu G-E, Mihai I-M, Bojin F,
Gavriliuc O, Paunescu V. The natural
adaptive
evolution of cancer: The metastatic ability of
cancer cells. Bosn J of Basic Med Sci
[Internet]. 2020Feb.3;. Available
from: https://www.bjbms.org/ojs/index.php/b
jbms/article/view/4565

12.^ Nguyen DX, Massagué J (May 2007).
"Genetic determinants of cancer
metastasis". Nature Reviews. Genetics. 8 (5):
341–52. doi:10.1038/nrg2101. PMID 17440531
. S2CID 17745552.

13.^ Zlotnik A, Burkhardt AM, Homey B
(August 2011). "Homeostatic chemokine
receptors and organ-specific
metastasis". Nature Reviews.
Immunology. 11 (9): 597–
606. doi:10.1038/nri3049. PMID 21866172. S2

CID 34438005.

14. ^ Drabsch Y, ten Dijke P (June 2011). "TGF- β signaling in breast cancer cell invasion and bone metastasis". Journal of Mammary Gland Biology and Neoplasia. 16 (2): 97–108. doi:10.1007/s10911-011-9217-1. PMC 309 5797. PMID 21494783.

15. ^ Yoshida BA, Sokoloff MM, Welch DR, Rinker-Schaeffer CW (November 2000). "Metastasis-suppressor genes: a review and perspective on an emerging field". Journal of the National Cancer Institute. 92 (21): 1717–30. doi:10.1093/jnci/92.21.1717. PMID 110586 15.

16. ^ Matteo Parri, Paola Chiarugi. "Rac and Rho GTPases in cancer cell motility control" 2010

17. ^ Friedl P, Wolf K (May 2003). "Tumour-cell invasion and migration: diversity and escape mechanisms". Nature Reviews. Cancer. 3 (5): 362–74. doi:10.1038/nrc1075. PMID 12724734 . S2CID 5547981.

18. ^ Escribano J, Chen MB, Moeendarbary E, Cao X, Shenoy V, Garcia-Aznar JM, et al. (May 2019). "Balance of mechanical forces drives endothelial gap formation and may facilitate cancer and immune-cell

extravasation". PLOS Computational Biology. 15 (5): e1006395. arXiv:1811.09326. Bibcode:2019PL SCB..15E6395E. doi:10.1371/journal.pcbi.1006395. PMC 6497229. PMID 31 048903.

19. ^ Weidner N, Semple JP, Welch WR, Folkman J (January 1991). "Tumor angiogenesis and metastasis--correlation in invasive breast carcinoma". The New England Journal of Medicine. 324 (1): 1–8. doi:10.1056/NEJM199101033240101. PMID 1701519.

20. ^ Gao D, Nolan DJ, Mellick AS, Bambino K, McDonnell K, Mittal V (January 2008). "Endothelial progenitor cells control the angiogenic switch in mouse lung metastasis". Science. 319 (5860): 195–8. Bibcode:2008Sci...319..195G. doi:10.1126/science.1150224. PMID 18187653. S2CID 1257 7022.

21. ^ Nolan DJ, Ciarrocchi A, Mellick AS, Jaggi JS, Bambino K, Gupta S, et al. (June 2007). "Bone marrow-derived endothelial progenitor cells are a major determinant of nascent tumor neovascularization". Genes & Development. 21 (12): 1546–58. doi:10.1101/gad.436307. PMC 1891431. P

MID 17575055.

22. ^ Mellick AS, Plummer PN, Nolan DJ, Gao D, Bambino K, Hahn M, et al. (September 2010). "Using the transcription factor inhibitor of DNA binding 1 to selectively target endothelial progenitor cells offers novel strategies to inhibit tumor angiogenesis and growth". Cancer Research. 70 (18): 7273–82. doi:10.1158/0008-5472.CAN-10-1142. PMC 3058751. PMID 20807818.

23. ^ Franci C, Zhou J, Jiang Z, Modrusan Z, Good Z, Jackson E, Kouros-Mehr H (2013). "Biomarkers of residual disease, disseminated tumor cells, and metastases in the MMTV-PyMT breast cancer model". PLOS ONE. 8 (3): e58183. Bibcode:2013PLoSO...858183F. doi:10.1371/journal.pone.0058183. PMC 3592916. PMID 23520493.

24. ^ Lujambio A, Esteller M (February 2009). "How epigenetics can explain human metastasis: a new role for microRNAs". Cell Cycle. 8 (3): 377–82. doi:10.4161/cc.8.3.7526. PMID 19177007.

25. ^ Ratnayake WS, Apostolatos AH, Ostrov DA, Acevedo-Duncan M (November 2017). "Two novel atypical PKC inhibitors;

ACPD and DNDA effectively mitigate cell proliferation and epithelial to mesenchymal transition of metastatic melanoma while inducing apoptosis". International Journal of Oncology. 51 (5): 1370–1382. doi:10.3892/ijo.2017.4131. PMC 564239 3. PMID 29048609.

26. ^ Jump up to:a b c Syn N, Wang L, Sethi G, Thiery JP, Goh BC (July 2016). "Exosome-Mediated Metastasis: From Epithelial-Mesenchymal Transition to Escape from Immunosurveillance". Trends in Pharmacological Sciences. 37 (7): 606–617. doi:10.1016/j.tips.2016.04.006. PMID 271 57716.

27. ^ List of included entries and references is found on main image page in Commons: Commons:File:Metastasis sites for common cancers.svg#Summary

28. ^ "Stephen Paget and the 'seed and soil' theory of metastatic dissemination", NIH

29. ^ Hart IR (1982). "'Seed and soil' revisited: mechanisms of site-specific metastasis". Cancer and Metastasis Reviews. 1 (1): 5–16. doi:10.1007/BF00049477. PMID 6764375. S2CID 19573769.

30. ^ Weinberg RA (2007). The Biology of

Cancer. New York: Taylor & Francis. ISBN 978-0-8153-4076-8. quoted in Angier N (3 April 2007). "Basics: A mutinous group of cells on a greedy, destructive task". The New York Times.

31. ^ Scott J, Kuhn P, Anderson AR (July 2012). "Unifying metastasis--integrating intravasation, circulation and end-organ colonization". Nature Reviews. Cancer. 12 (7): 445–6. doi:10.1038/nrc3287. PMC 4533867. PMID 22912952.

32. ^ Ettinger DS, Agulnik M, Cates JM, Cristea M, Denlinger CS, Eaton KD, et al. (December 2011). "NCCN Clinical Practice Guidelines Occult primary". Journal of the National Comprehensive Cancer Network. 9 (12): 1358–95. doi:10.6004/jnccn.2011.0117. PMID 22157556.

33. ^ Jump up to:a b Briasoulis E, Pavlidis N (1997). "Cancer of Unknown Primary Origin". The Oncologist. 2 (3): 142–152. doi:10.1634/theoncologist.2-3-142. PMID 10388044.

34.^ Poste G, Fidler IJ (January 1980). "The pathogenesis of cancer metastasis". Nature. 283 (5743): 139–46. Bibcode:1980Natur.283..139P. CiteSeerX

10.1.1.553.5472. doi:10.1038/283139a0. PMID 6985715. S2CID 4302076.

35. ^ Jump up to:a b c d e f Ramaswamy S, Ross KN, Lander ES, Golub TR (January 2003). "A molecular signature of metastasis in primary solid tumors". Nature Genetics. 33 (1): 49–54. doi:10.1038/ng1060. PMID 12469122. S2CID 12059602.

36. ^ van 't Veer LJ, Dai H, van de Vijver MJ, He YD, Hart AA, Mao M, et al. (January 2002). "Gene expression profiling predicts clinical outcome of breast cancer". Nature. 415 (6871): 530–6. doi:10.1038/415530a. hdl:1874/15552. PMID 11823860. S2CID 4369266.

37. ^ Bakhoum SF, Ngo B, Laughney AM, Cavallo JA, Murphy CJ, Ly P, et al. (January 2018). "Chromosomal instability drives metastasis through a cytosolic DNA response". Nature. 553 (7689): 467–472. Bibcode:2018Natur.553..467B. doi:10.1038/nature25432. PMC 5785464. PMID 29342134.

38. ^ Irwin KE, Greer JA, Khatib J, Temel JS, Pirl WF (February 2013). "Early palliative care and metastatic non-small cell lung cancer: potential mechanisms of prolonged

survival". Chronic Respiratory Disease. 10 (1): 35–47. doi:10.1177/1479972312471549. PMID 233 55404. S2CID 6743524.

39. ^ Garsa A, Jang JK, Baxi S, Chen C, Akinniranye O, Hall O, et al. (2021). "Radiation Therapy for Brain Metastases: A Systematic Review". Practical Radiation Oncology. 11 (5): 354–365. doi:10.1016/j.prro.2021.04.002. PMID 341 19447.

40. ^ Shahriyari L (2016). "A new hypothesis: some metastases are the result of inflammatory processes by adapted cells, especially adapted immune cells at sites of inflammation". F1000Research. 5: 175. doi:10.12688/f1000research.8055.1. PMC 4847566. PMID 27158448.

41. ^ López-Lázaro M (2015-01-01). "The migration ability of stem cells can explain the existence of cancer of unknown primary site. Rethinking metastasis". Oncoscience. 2 (5): 467–75. doi:10.18632/oncoscience.159. PMC 4468 332. PMID 26097879.

42. ^ Jump up to:a b Sarna M, Krzykawska-Serda M, Jakubowska M, Zadlo A, Urbanska K (June 2019). "Melanin presence inhibits

melanoma cell spread in mice in a unique mechanical fashion". Scientific Reports. 9 (1): 9280. Bibcode:2019NatSR. 9.9280S. doi:10.1 038/s41598-019-45643-9. PMC 6594928. PMID 31243305.

43. ^ Kelland K (17 March 2014). "Archaeologists discover earliest example of human with cancer". Reuters. Retrieved 18 March 2014.
44. ^ Ghosh P (18 March 2014). "Ancient skeleton is the earliest case of cancer yet detected". BBC. Retrieved 18 March 2014.
45. ^ Ross P (17 March 2014). "Possible Oldest Cancer Found In 3,000-Year-Old Skeleton Could Reveal 'Evolution' Of Modern Disease". International Business Times. Retrieved 18 March 2014.

External links[edit]

Q&A: Metastatic Cancer—from the National Cancer Institute
· How does cancer spread - the route by TED-Ed
D
· MeSH: D00

Overview of tumors, cancer and oncology

Conditions		
	Benign tumors	· Hyperplasia · Cyst · Pseudocyst · Hamartoma
	Malignant progression	· Dysplasia · Carcinoma in situ · Cancer · Metastasis · Primary tumor · Sentinel lymph node
	Topography	· Head and neck (oral, nasopharyngeal) · Digestive system · Respiratory system · Bone

Histology		· Skin
		· Blood
		· Urogenital
		· Nervous system
		· Endocrine system
		· Carcinoma
		· Sarcoma
		· Blastoma
		· Papilloma
		· Adenoma
Other		· Precancerous condition
		· Paraneoplastic syndrome
Staging/		· TNM
		· Ann Arbor
	grading	Carcinog enesis

- ading system
- Dukes classification
- Clonally transm
- issible cancer
- Carcinogenic bact
- eria
- Misc. Research

239

What Is Cancer?

ON THIS
PAGE
- The Definition of Cancer
- Differences between Cancer Cells and Normal Cells
- How Does Cancer Develop?
- Types of Genes that Cause Cancer
- When Cancer Spreads 240

- Tissue Changes that Are Not Cancer
- Types of Cancer
'

The
Definition
of Cancer
Cancer is a
disease in
which
some of
the body's
cells grow

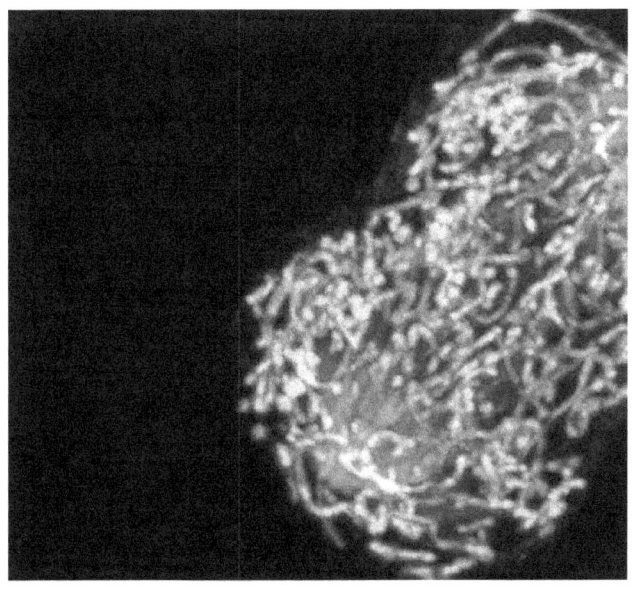

A dividing breast cancer cell.
Credit: National Cancer Institute / Univ. of Pittsburgh Cancer Institute

uncontrollably and spread to other parts of the body.
Cancer can start almost anywhere in the human body, which is made up of trillions of cells. Normally, human cells grow and multiply (through a process called cell division) to form new cells as the body needs them. When cells grow old or become damaged, they die, and new cells take their place.
Sometimes this orderly process breaks down, and abnormal or damaged cells grow

and multiply when they shouldn't. These cells may form tumors, which are lumps of tissue. Tumors can be cancerous or not cancerous (benign).

Cancerous tumors spread into, or invade, nearby tissues and can travel to distant places in the body to form new tumors (a process called metastasis). Cancerous tumors may also be called malignant tumors. Many cancers form solid tumors, but cancers of the blood, such as leukemias, generally do not.

Benign tumors do not spread into, or invade, nearby tissues. When removed, benign tumors usually don't grow back, whereas cancerous tumors sometimes do. Benign tumors can sometimes be quite large, however. Some can cause serious symptoms or be life threatening, such as benign tumors in the brain.

Differences between Cancer Cells and Normal Cells

Cancer cells differ from normal cells in many ways. For instance, cancer cells:

· grow in the absence of signals telling them to grow. Normal cells only grow when they receive such signals.

· ignore signals that normally tell cells to stop

dividing or to die (a process known as programmed cell death, or apoptosis).

- invade into nearby areas and spread to other areas of the body. Normal cells stop growing when they encounter other cells, and most normal cells do not move around the body.
- tell blood vessels to grow toward tumors. These blood vessels supply tumors with oxygen and nutrients and remove waste products from tumors.
- hide from the immune system. The immune system normally eliminates damaged or abnormal cells.
- trick the immune system into helping cancer cells stay alive and grow. For instance, some cancer cells convince immune cells to protect the tumor instead of attacking it.
- accumulate multiple changes in their chromosomes, such as duplications and deletions of chromosome parts. Some cancer cells have double the normal number of chromosomes.
- rely on different kinds of nutrients than normal cells. In addition, some cancer cells make energy from nutrients in a different way than most normal cells. This lets cancer cells grow more quickly.

Many times, cancer cells rely so heavily on

these abnormal behaviors that they can't survive without them. Researchers have taken advantage of this fact, developing therapies that target the abnormal features of cancer cells. For example, some cancer therapies prevent blood vessels from growing toward tumors, essentially starving the tumor of needed nutrients.

How Does Cancer Develop?

Cancer is a genetic disease—that is, it is caused by changes to genes that control the way our cells function,

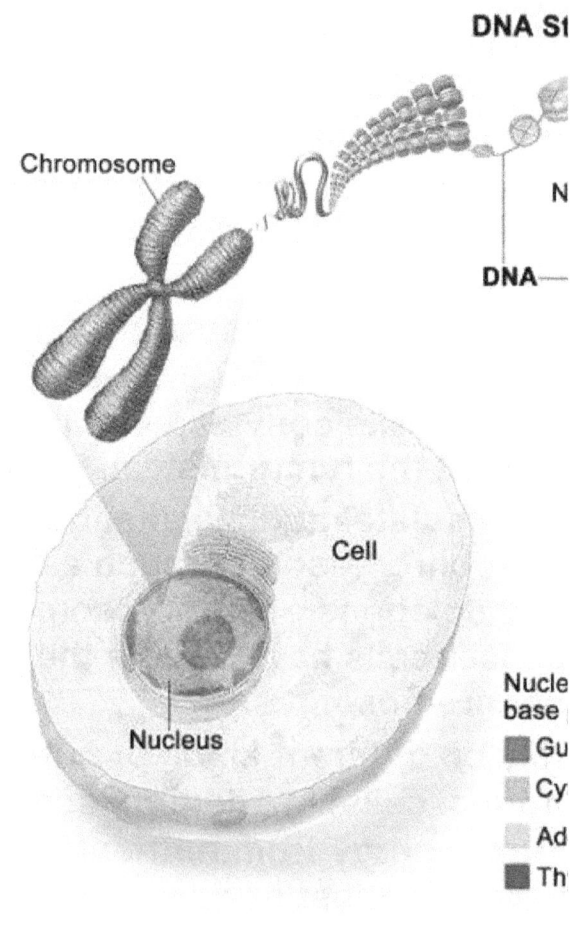

DNA St

Chromosome

N

DNA

Cell

Nucle
base

Nucleus

Gu

Cy

Ad

Th

Cancer is caused by certain changes to genes, the basic physical units of inheritance. Genes are arranged in long strands of tightly packed DNA called chromosomes.

Credit: © Terese Winslow

especially how they grow and divide. Genetic changes that cause cancer can happen because:

- of errors that occur as cells divide.
- of damage to DNA caused by harmful substances in the environment, such as the chemicals in tobacco smoke and ultraviolet rays from the sun. (Our Cancer Causes and Prevention section has more information.)
- they were inherited from our parents. The body normally eliminates cells with damaged DNA before they turn cancerous. But the body's ability to do so goes down as we age. This is part of the reason why there is a higher risk of cancer later in life. Each person's cancer has a unique combination of genetic changes. As the cancer continues to grow, additional changes will occur. Even within the same tumor, different cells may have different genetic changes.

Fundamentals of Cancer
Previous

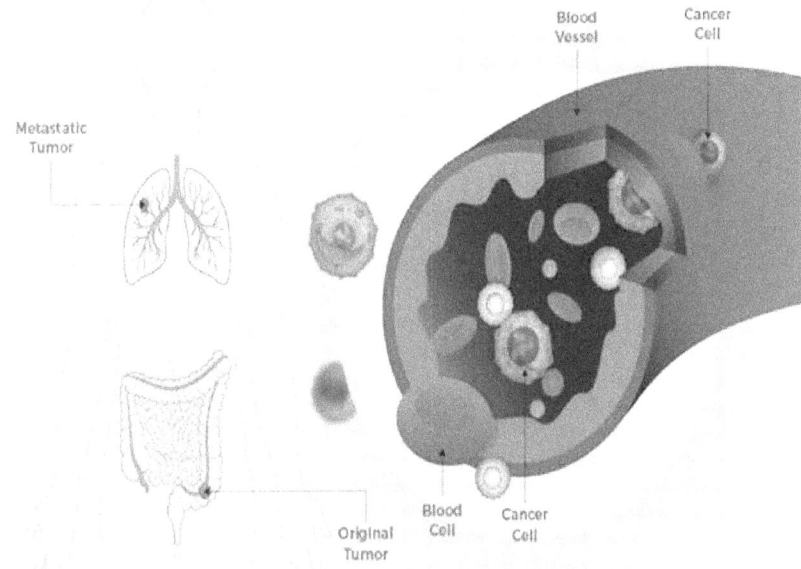

Cancer cells can break away from the original tumor and travel through the blood or lymph system to distant locations in the body, where they exit the vessels to form additional tumors. This is called metastasis.

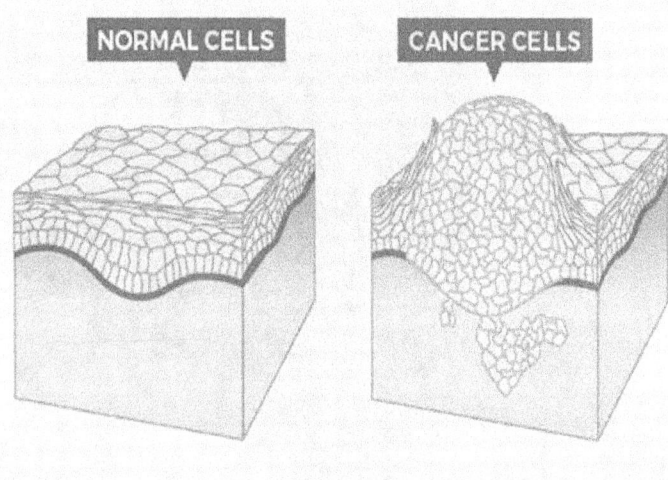

Cancer is a disease caused when cells divide uncontrollably and spread into surrounding tissues.

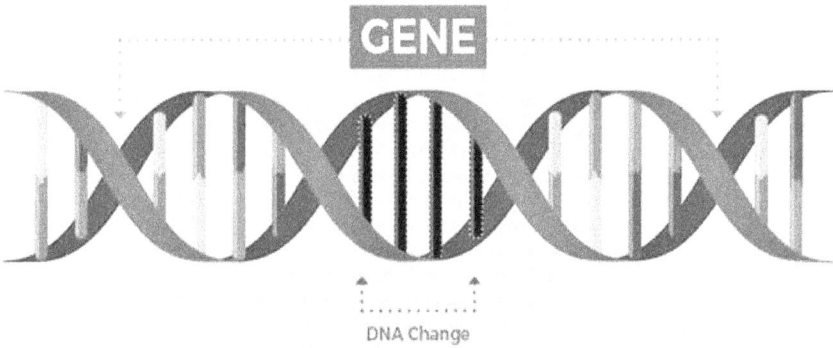

DNA Change

Cancer is caused by changes to DNA. Most cancer-causing DNA changes occur in sections of DNA called genes. These changes are also called genetic changes.

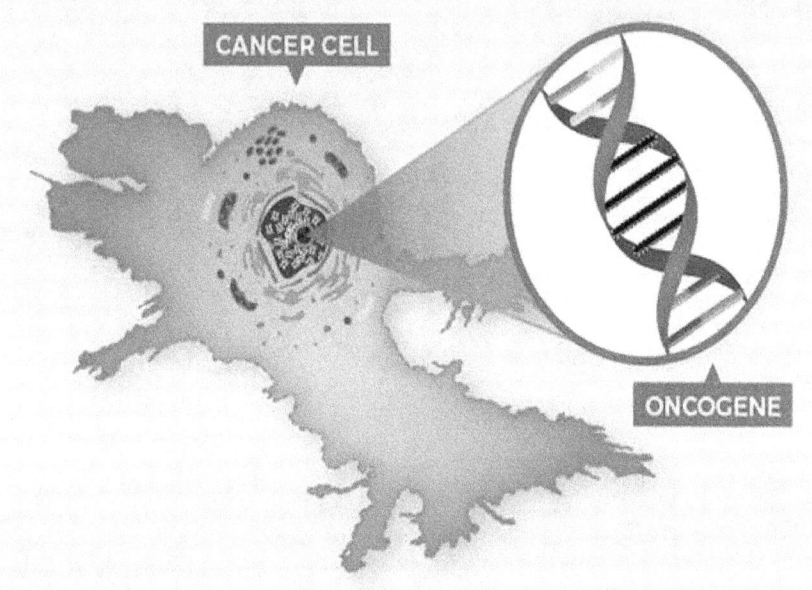

A DNA change can cause genes involved in normal cell growth to become oncogenes. Unlike normal genes, oncogenes cannot be turned off, so they cause uncontrolled cell growth.

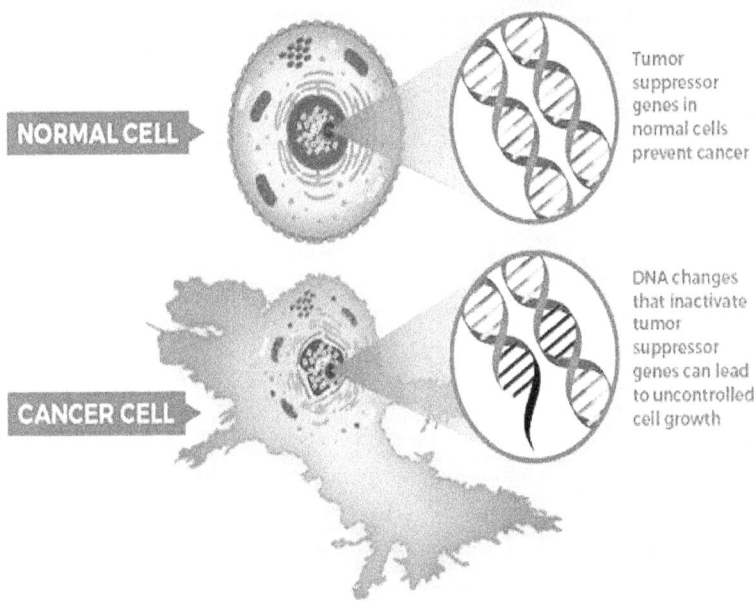

NORMAL CELL

Tumor suppressor genes in normal cells prevent cancer

CANCER CELL

DNA changes that inactivate tumor suppressor genes can lead to uncontrolled cell growth

In normal cells, tumor suppressor genes prevent cancer by slowing or stopping cell growth. DNA changes that inactivate tumor suppressor genes can lead to uncontrolled cell growth and cancer.

251

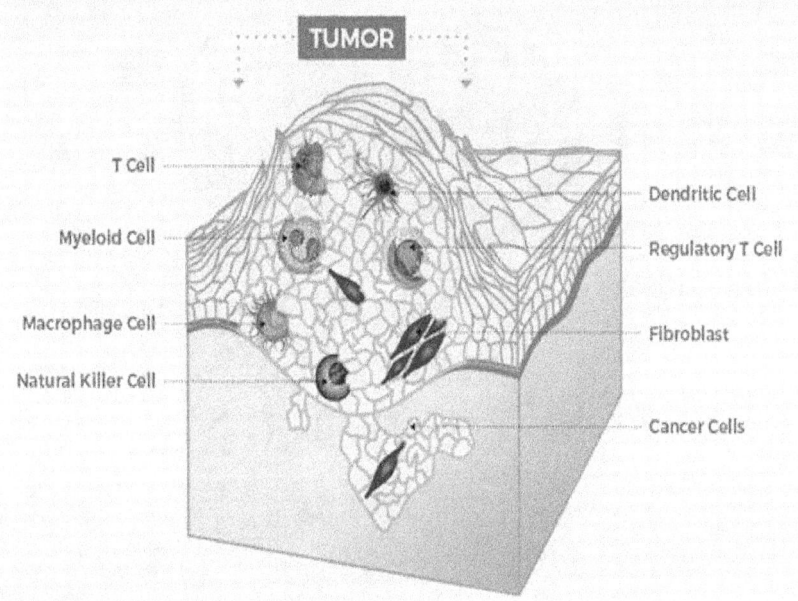

Within a tumor, cancer cells are surrounded by a variety of immune cells, fibroblasts, molecules, and blood vessels—what's known as the tumor microenvironment. Cancer cells can change the microenvironment, which in turn can affect how cancer grows and spreads.

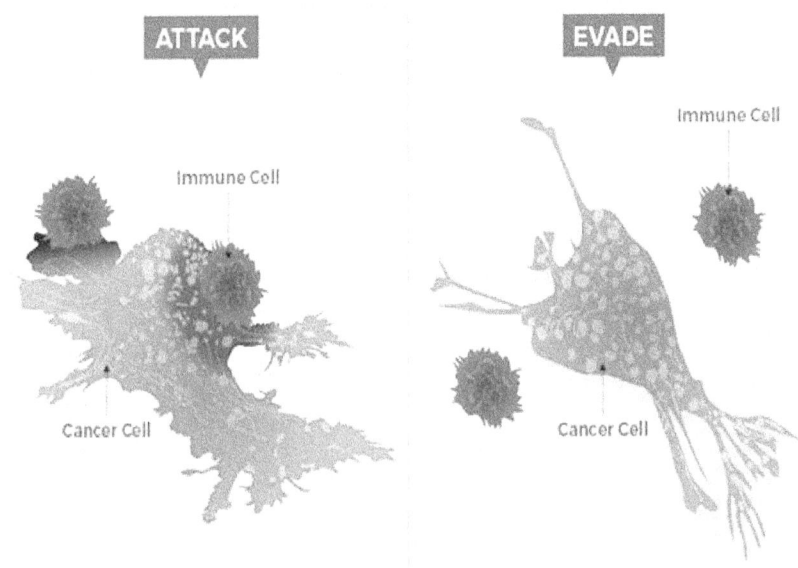

Immune system cells can detect and attack cancer cells. But some cancer cells can avoid detection or thwart an attack. Some cancer treatments can help the immune system better detect and kill cancer cells.

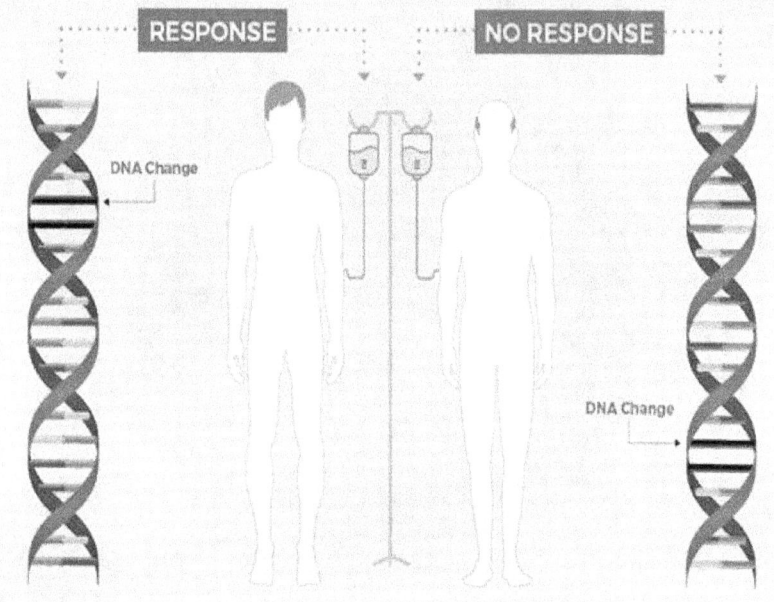

Each person's cancer has a unique combination of genetic changes. Specific genetic changes may make a person's cancer more or less likely to respond to certain treatments.

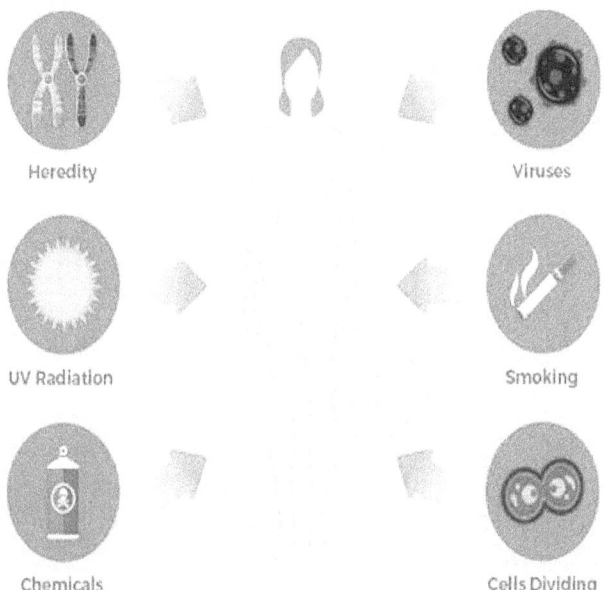

Heredity

Viruses

UV Radiation

Smoking

Chemicals

Cells Dividing

Genetic changes that cause cancer can be inherited or arise from certain environmental exposures. Genetic changes can also happen because of errors that occur as cells divide.

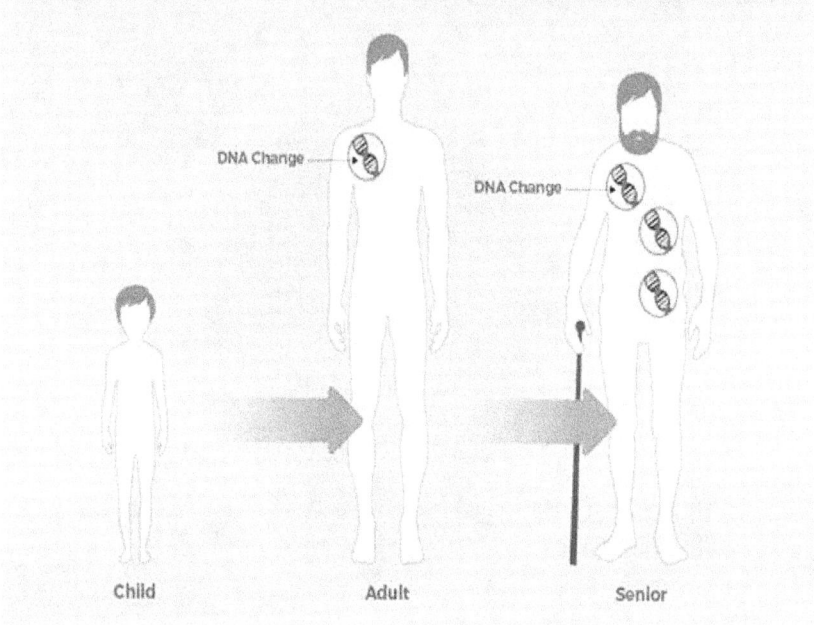

Most often, cancer-causing genetic changes accumulate slowly as a person ages, leading to a higher risk of cancer later in life.

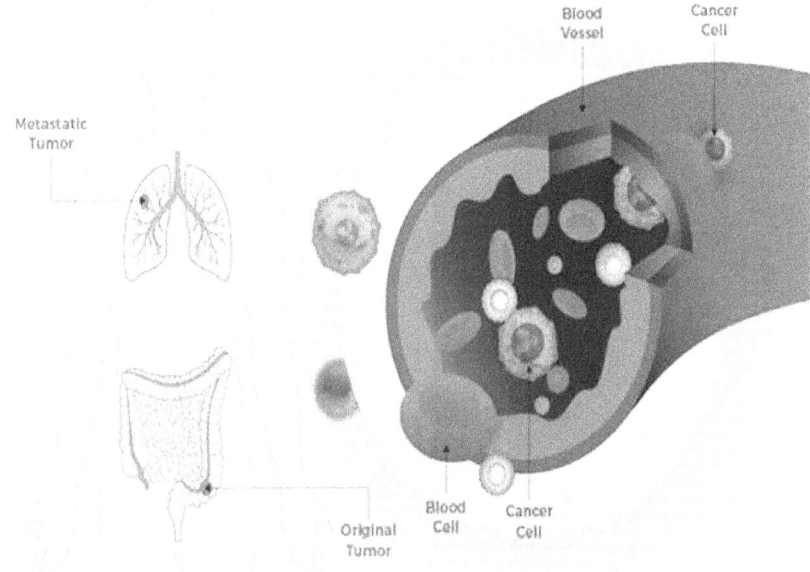

Cancer cells can break away from the original tumor and travel through the blood or lymph system to distant locations in the body, where they exit the vessels to form additional tumors. This is called metastasis.

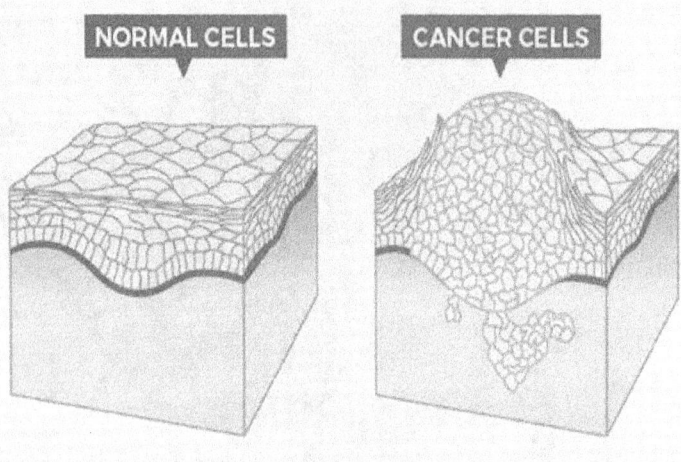

NORMAL CELLS

CANCER CELLS

Cancer is a disease caused when cells divide uncontrollably and spread into surrounding tissues.

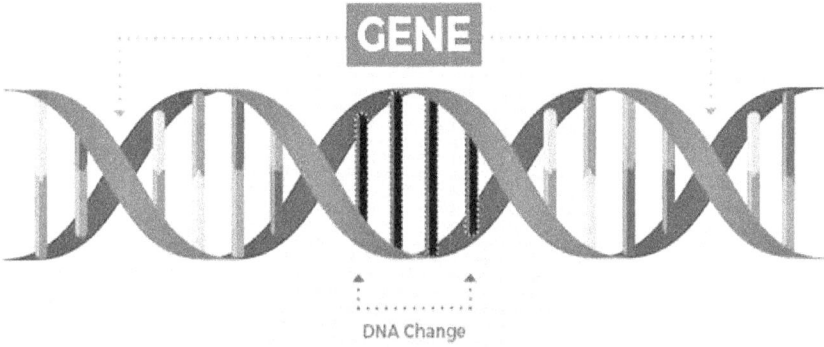

DNA Change

Cancer is caused by changes to DNA. Most cancer-causing DNA changes occur in sections of DNA called genes. These changes are also called genetic changes.

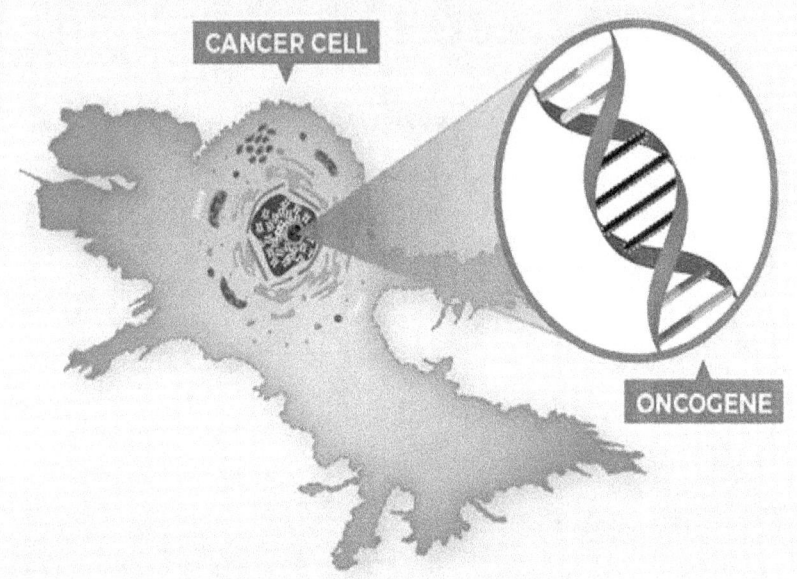

CANCER CELL

ONCOGENE

A DNA change can cause genes involved in normal cell growth to become oncogenes. Unlike normal genes, oncogenes cannot be turned off, so they cause uncontrolled cell growth.

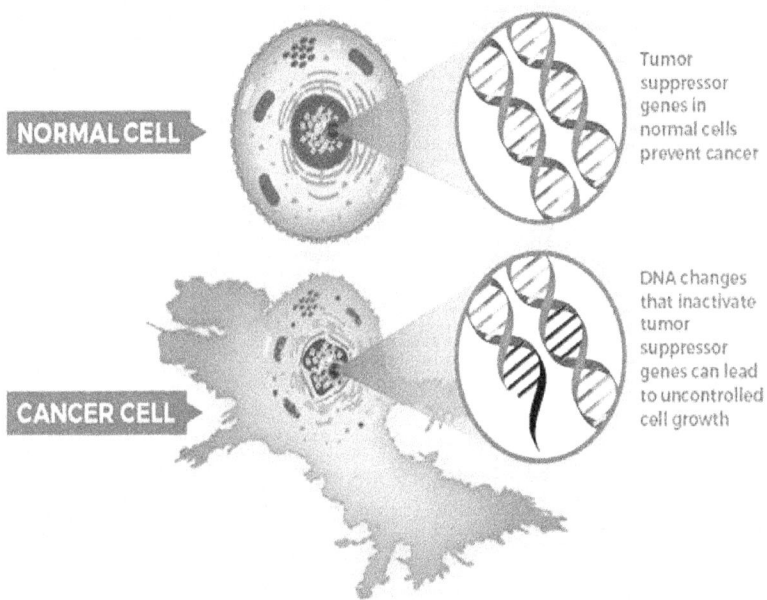

Tumor suppressor genes in normal cells prevent cancer

NORMAL CELL

DNA changes that inactivate tumor suppressor genes can lead to uncontrolled cell growth

CANCER CELL

In normal cells, tumor suppressor genes prevent cancer by slowing or stopping cell growth. DNA changes that inactivate tumor suppressor genes can lead to uncontrolled cell growth and cancer.

261

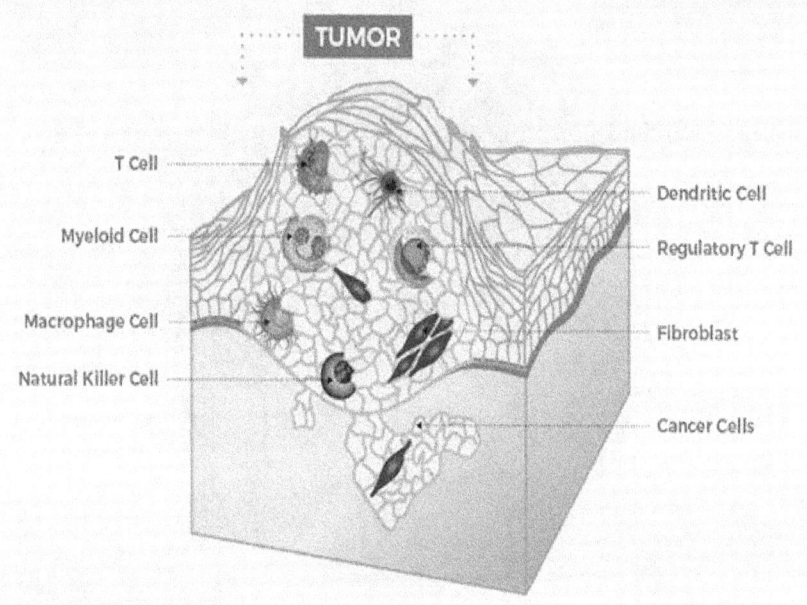

Within a tumor, cancer cells are surrounded by a variety of immune cells, fibroblasts, molecules, and blood vessels—what's known as the tumor microenvironment. Cancer cells can change the microenvironment, which in turn can affect how cancer grows and spreads.

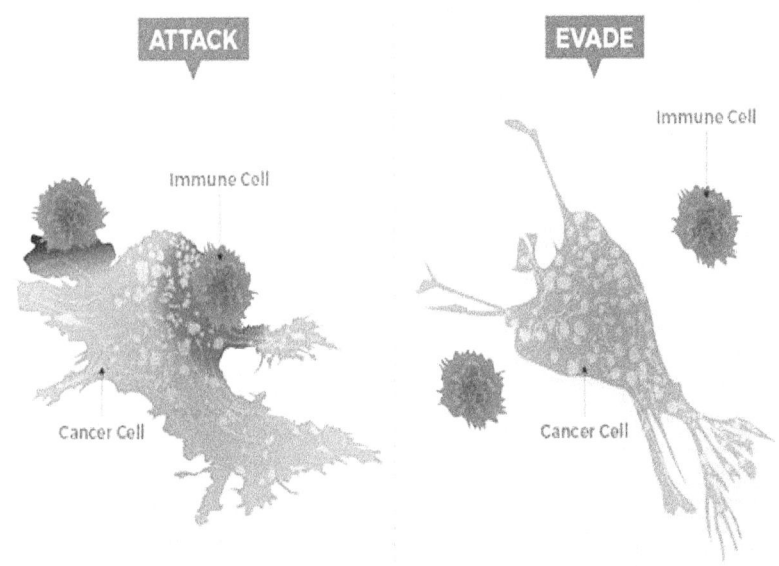

ATTACK

EVADE

Immune Cell

Immune Cell

Cancer Cell

Cancer Cell

Immune system cells can detect and attack cancer cells. But some cancer cells can avoid detection or thwart an attack. Some cancer treatments can help the immune system better detect and kill cancer cells.

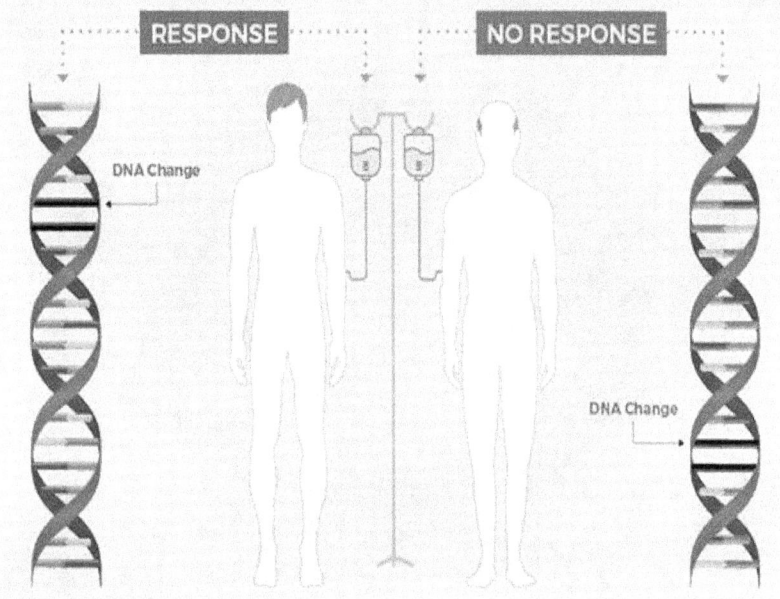

Each person's cancer has a unique combination of genetic changes. Specific genetic changes may make a person's cancer more or less likely to respond to certain treatments.

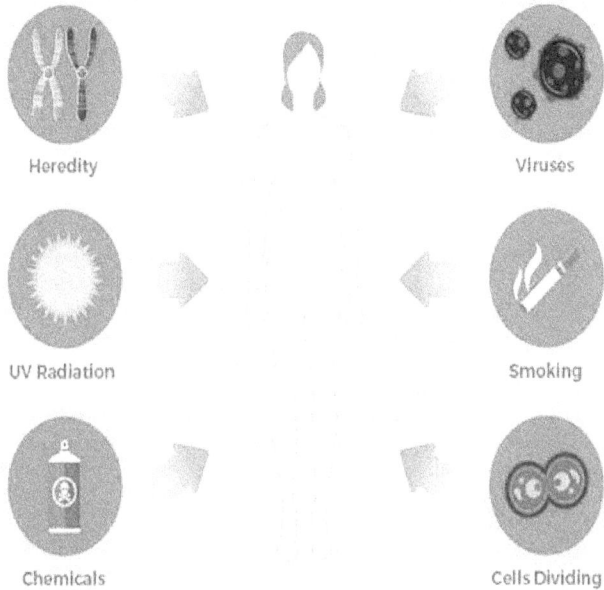

Heredity

Viruses

UV Radiation

Smoking

Chemicals

Cells Dividing

Genetic changes that cause cancer can be inherited or arise from certain environmental exposures. Genetic changes can also happen because of errors that occur as cells divide.

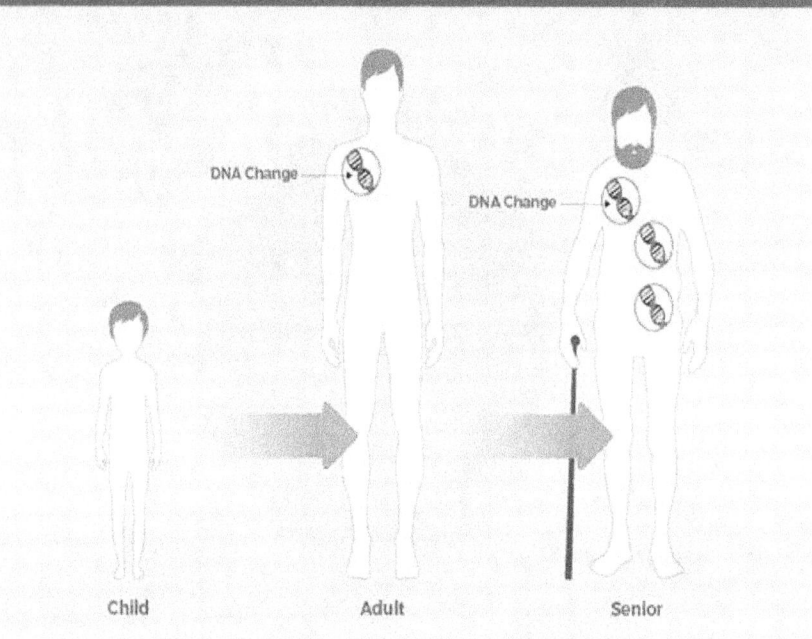

Most often, cancer-causing genetic changes accumulate slowly as a person ages, leading to a higher risk of cancer later in life.

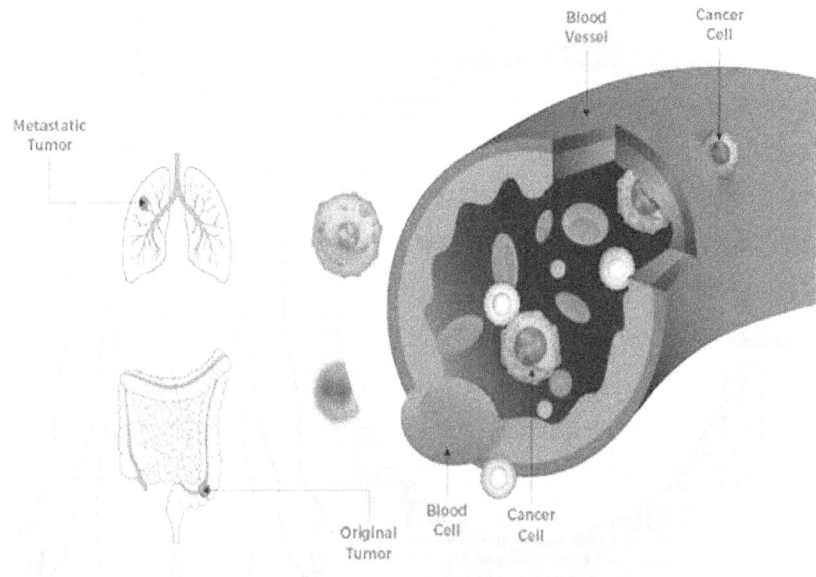

Cancer cells can break away from the original tumor and travel through the blood or lymph system to distant locations in the body, where they exit the vessels to form additional tumors. This is called metastasis. Next

1/10

Types of Genes
that Cause Cancer
The genetic changes that contribute to cancer tend to affect three main types of genes—proto-oncogenes, tumor suppressor

genes, and DNA repair genes. These changes are sometimes called "drivers" of cancer.

Proto-oncogenes are involved in normal cell growth and division. However, when these genes are altered in certain ways or are more active than normal, they may become cancer-causing genes (or oncogenes), allowing cells to grow and survive when they should not.

Tumor suppressor genes are also involved in controlling cell growth and division. Cells with certain alterations in tumor suppressor genes may divide in an uncontrolled manner. DNA repair genes are involved in fixing damaged DNA. Cells with mutations in these genes tend to develop additional mutations in other genes and changes in their chromosomes, such as duplications and deletions of chromosome parts. Together, these mutations may cause the cells to become cancerous.

As scientists have learned more about the molecular changes that lead to cancer, they have found that certain mutations commonly occur in many types of cancer. Now there are many cancer treatments available that target gene mutations found in cancer.

A few of these treatments can be used by anyone with a cancer that has the targeted mutation, no matter where the cancer started growing. When Cancer Spreads A cancer that has spread from the place where it first formed to another place in the

Cancer spreads to other parts of the body

Liver metastasis

Primary cancer

In metastasis, cancer cells break away from where they first formed and form new tumors in other parts of the body.
Credit: © Terese Winslow

body is called metastatic cancer. The process by which cancer cells spread to other parts of the body is called metastasis. Metastatic cancer has the same name and the same type of cancer cells as the original, or primary, cancer. For example, breast cancer that forms a metastatic tumor in the lung is metastatic breast cancer, not lung cancer.

Under a microscope, metastatic cancer cells generally look the same as cells of the original cancer. Moreover, metastatic cancer cells and cells of the original cancer usually have some molecular features in common, such as the presence of specific chromosome changes.

In some cases, treatment may help prolong the lives of people with metastatic cancer. In other cases, the primary goal of treatment for metastatic cancer is to control the growth of the cancer or to relieve symptoms it is causing. Metastatic tumors can cause severe damage to how the body functions, and most people who die of cancer die of metastatic disease.

Tissue Changes that Are Not Cancer

Not every change in the body's tissues is cancer. Some tissue changes may develop into cancer if they are not treated, however. Here are some examples of tissue changes that are not cancer but, in some cases, are monitored because they could become cancer:

- Hyperplasia occurs when cells within a tissue multiply faster than normal and extra cells build up. However, the cells and the way the tissue is organized still look normal under a microscope. Hyperplasia can be caused by several factors or conditions, including chronic irritation.

- Dysplasia is a more advanced condition than hyperplasia. In dysplasia, there is also a buildup of extra cells. But the cells look abnormal and there are changes in how the tissue is organized. In general, the more abnormal the cells and tissue look, the greater the chance that cancer will form. Some types of dysplasia may need to be monitored or treated, but others do not. An example of dysplasia is an abnormal mole (called a dysplastic nevus) that forms on the skin. A dysplastic nevus can turn into melanoma, although most do not.

- Carcinoma in situ is an even more advanced condition. Although it is sometimes called stage 0 cancer, it is not cancer because the abnormal cells do not invade nearby tissue the way that cancer cells do. But because some carcinomas in situ may become cancer, they are usually treated.

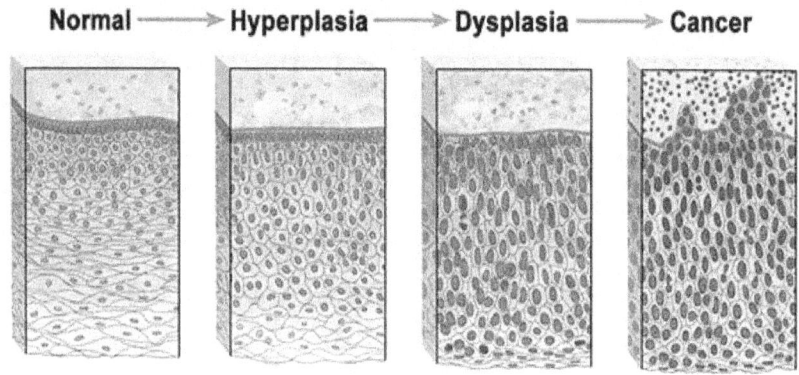

Normal ——→ Hyperplasia ——→ Dysplasia ——→ Cancer

© 2014 Terese Winslow LLC
U.S. Govt. has certain rights

Normal cells may become cancer cells. Before cancer cells form in tissues of the body, the cells go through abnormal changes called hyperplasia and dysplasia. In hyperplasia, there is an increase in the number of cells in an organ or tissue that appear normal under a microscope. In dysplasia, the cells look abnormal under a microscope but are not cancer. Hyperplasia and dysplasia may or may not become cancer.
Credit: © Terese Winslow
Types of Cancer
There are more than 100 types of cancer.

Types of cancer are usually named for the organs or tissues where the cancers form. For example, lung cancer starts in the lung, and brain cancer starts in the brain. Cancers also may be described by the type of cell that formed them, such as an epithelial cell or a squamous cell.

You can search NCI's website for information on specific types of cancer based on the cancer's location in the body or by using our A to Z List of Cancers. We also have information on childhood cancers and cancers in adolescents and young adults.

Here are some categories of cancers that begin in specific types of cells:

Carcinoma

Carcinomas are the most common type of cancer. They are formed by epithelial cells, which are the cells that cover the inside and outside surfaces of the body. There are many types of epithelial cells, which often have a column-like shape when viewed under a microscope.

Carcinomas that begin in different epithelial cell types have specific names:

Adenocarcinoma is a cancer that forms in epithelial cells that produce fluids or mucus.

Tissues with this type of epithelial cell are sometimes called glandular tissues. Most cancers of the breast, colon, and prostate are adenocarcinomas.

Basal cell carcinoma is a cancer that begins in the lower or basal (base) layer of the epidermis, which is a person's outer layer of skin.

Squamous cell carcinoma is a cancer that forms in squamous cells, which are epithelial cells that lie just beneath the outer surface of the skin. Squamous cells also line many other organs, including the stomach, intestines, lungs, bladder, and kidneys. Squamous cells look flat, like fish scales, when viewed under a microscope. Squamous cell carcinomas are sometimes called epidermoid carcinomas.

Transitional cell carcinoma is a cancer that forms in a type of epithelial tissue called transitional epithelium, or urothelium. This tissue, which is made up of many layers of epithelial cells that can get bigger and smaller, is found in the linings of the bladder, ureters, and part of the kidneys (renal pelvis), and a few other organs. Some cancers of the bladder, ureters, and kidneys are transitional cell carcinomas.

Sarcoma

Sarcomas are cancers that form in bone and soft tissues, including muscle, fat, blood vessels, ly mph vessels, and fibrous tissue (such as tendons and ligaments).

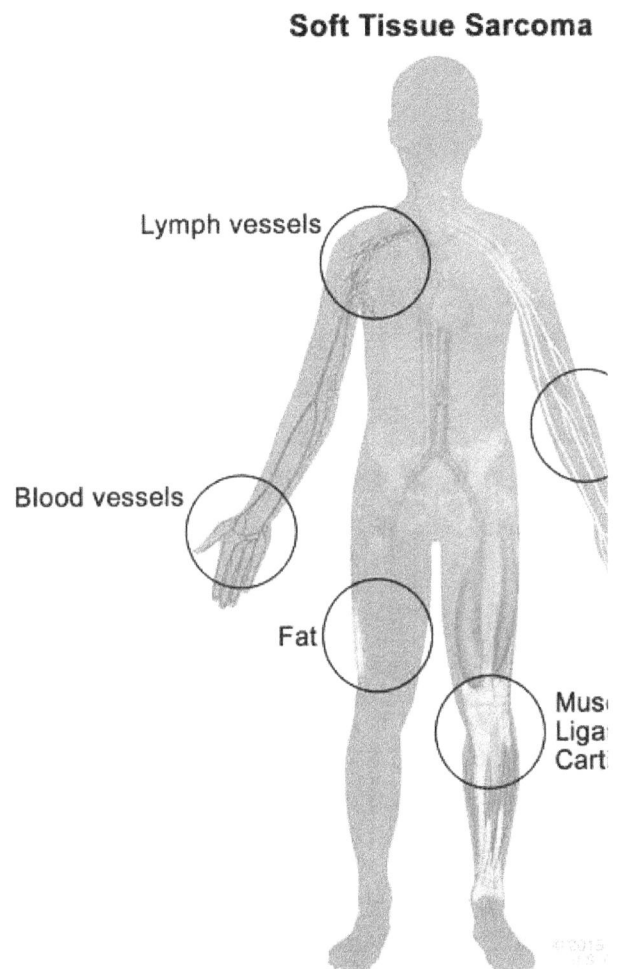

Soft Tissue Sarcoma

Lymph vessels

Blood vessels

Fat

Mus
Liga
Cart

Soft tissue sarcoma forms in soft tissues of the body, including muscle, tendons, fat, blood vessels, lymph vessels, nerves, and tissue around joints.
Credit: © Terese Winslow

Osteosarcoma is the most common cancer of bone. The most common types of soft tissue sarcoma are leiomyosarcoma, Kaposi

275

sarcoma, malignant fibrous histiocytoma, liposarcoma, and dermatofibrosarcoma protuberans. Our page on soft tissue sarcoma has more information.

Leukemia

Cancers that begin in the blood-forming tissue of the bone marrow are called leukemias. These cancers do not form solid tumors. Instead, large numbers of abnormal white blood cells (leukemia cells and leukemic blast cells) build up in the blood and bone marrow, crowding out normal blood cells. The low level of normal blood cells can make it harder for the body to get oxygen to its tissues, control bleeding, or fight infections.

There are four common types of leukemia, which are grouped based on how quickly the disease gets worse (acute or chronic) and on the type of blood cell the cancer starts in (lymphoblastic or myeloid). Acute forms of leukemia grow quickly and chronic forms grow more slowly.

Our page on leukemia has more information.

Lymphoma

Lymphoma is cancer that begins in lymphocytes (T cells or B cells). These are disease-fighting white blood cells that are part of the immune system. In lymphoma, abnormal lymphocytes build up in lymph nodes and lymph vessels, as well as in other organs of the body.

There are two main types of lymphoma:

Hodgkin lymphoma – People with this disease have abnormal lymphocytes that are called Reed-Sternberg cells. These cells usually form from B cells.

Non-Hodgkin lymphoma – This is a large group of cancers that start in lymphocytes. The cancers can grow quickly or slowly and can form from B cells or T cells.

Our page on lymphoma has more information.

Multiple Myeloma

Multiple myeloma is cancer that begins in plasma cells, another type of immune cell. The abnormal plasma cells, called myeloma cells, build up in the bone marrow and form tumors in bones all through the body.

Multiple myeloma is also called plasma cell myeloma and Kahler disease.

Our page on multiple myeloma and other plasma cell neoplasms has more information.

Melanoma

Melanoma is cancer that begins in cells that become melanocytes, which are specialized cells that make melanin (the pigment that gives skin its color). Most melanomas form on the skin, but melanomas can also form in other pigmented tissues, such as the eye. Our pages on skin cancer and intraocular melanoma have more information.

Brain and Spinal Cord Tumors

There are different types of brain and spinal cord tumors. These tumors are named based on the type of cell in which they formed and where the tumor first formed in the central nervous system. For example, an astrocytic tumor begins in star-shaped brain cells called astrocytes, which help keep nerve cells healthy. Brain tumors can be benign (not cancer) or malignant (cancer). Our pages on brain and spinal cord tumors in adults and brain and spinal cord tumors in children have more information.

Other Types of

Tumors Germ Cell

Tumors

Germ cell tumors are a type of tumor that begins in the cells that give rise to sperm or eggs. These tumors can occur almost anywhere in the body and can be either benign or malignant.

Our page of cancers by body location/system includes a list of germ cell tumors with links to more information.

Neuroendocrine Tumors

Neuroendocrine tumors form from cells that release hormones into the blood in response to a signal from the nervous system. These tumors, which may make higher-than-normal amounts of hormones, can cause many different symptoms. Neuroendocrine tumors may be benign or malignant.

Our definition of neuroendocrine tumors has more information.

Carcinoid Tumors

Carcinoid tumors are a type of neuroendocrine tumor. They are slow-growing tumors that are usually found in the gastrointestinal system (most often in the rectum and small intestine). Carcinoid tumors may spread to the liver or other sites in the body, and they may secrete substances such as serotonin or prostaglandins, causing carcinoid syndrome.

Breast cancer is the most common type of cancer in the UK. Most women diagnosed with breast cancer are over the age of 50, but younger women can also get breast cancer.

About 1 in 8 women are diagnosed with breast cancer during their lifetime. There's a good chance of recovery if it's detected at an early stage.

For this reason, it's vital that women check their breasts regularly for any changes and always have any changes examined by a GP. In rare cases, men can also be diagnosed with breast cancer. Find out more about breast cancer in men.

Symptoms of breast cancer

Breast cancer can have several symptoms, but the first noticeable symptom is usually a lump or area of thickened breast tissue.

Most breast lumps are not cancerous, but it's always best to have them checked by a doctor.

You should also see a GP if you notice any of these symptoms:

- a change in the size or shape of one or both breasts
- discharge from either of your nipples, which may be streaked with blood
- a lump or swelling in either of your armpits
- dimpling on the skin of your breasts
- a rash on or around your nipple

- a change in the appearance of your nipple, such as becoming sunken into your breast

Breast pain is not usually a symptom of breast cancer.

Find out more about the symptoms of breast cancer.

Causes of breast cancer

The exact causes of breast cancer are not fully understood. However, there are certain factors known to increase the risk of breast cancer.

These include:

- age – the risk increases as you get older
- a family history of breast cancer
- a previous diagnosis of breast cancer
- a previous non-cancerous (benign) breast lump
- being tall, overweight or obese
- drinking alcohol

Find out more about the causes of breast cancer.

Diagnosing breast cancer

After examining your breasts, a GP may refer you to a specialist breast cancer clinic for further tests. This might include breast screening (mammography) or taking a small sample of breast tissue to be examined

under a microscope (a biopsy).
Find out more about how breast cancer is diagnosed.

Types of breast cancer

There are several different types of breast cancer, which develop in different parts of the breast.

Breast cancer is often divided into either:

- non-invasive breast cancer (carcinoma in situ) – found in the ducts of the breast (ductal carcinoma in situ, or DCIS) which has not spread into the breast tissue surrounding the ducts. Non-invasive breast cancer is usually found during a mammogram and rarely shows as a breast lump.
- invasive breast cancer – where the cancer cells have spread through the lining of the ducts into the surrounding breast tissue. This is the most common type of breast cancer.

Other, less common types of breast cancer include:

- invasive (and pre-invasive) lobular breast cancer
- inflammatory breast cancer
- Paget's disease of the breast

It's possible for breast cancer to spread to

other parts of the body, usually through the blood or the axillary lymph nodes. These are small lymphatic glands that filter bacteria and cells from the mammary gland.
If this happens, it's known as secondary, or metastatic, breast cancer.
Breast cancer screening
Mammographic screening, where X-ray images of the breast are taken, is the most commonly available way of finding a change in your breast tissue (lesion) at an early stage.
However, you should be aware that a mammogram might fail to detect some breast cancers.
It might also increase your chances of having extra tests and interventions, including surgery, even if you're not affected by breast cancer.
Women with a higher-than-average risk of developing breast cancer may be offered screening and genetic testing for the condition.
As the risk of breast cancer increases with age, all women who are 50 to 70 years old are invited for breast cancer screening every 3 years.
Women over the age of 70 are also entitled

to screening and can arrange an appointment through their GP or local screening unit.

The NHS is in the process of extending the programme as a trial, offering screening to some women aged 47 to 73.

Find out more about breast cancer screening.

Find a breast cancer screening services near you

Treating breast cancer

If cancer is detected at an early stage, it can be treated before it spreads to other parts of the body.

Breast cancer is treated using a combination of:

- surgery
- chemotherapy
- radiotherapy

Surgery is usually the first type of treatment you'll have, followed by chemotherapy or radiotherapy or, in some cases, hormone or targeted treatments.

The type of surgery and the treatment you have afterwards will depend on the type of breast cancer you have. Your doctor should discuss the best treatment plan with you.

In a small proportion of women, breast

cancer is discovered after it's spread to other parts of the body (metastatic breast cancer).

Secondary cancer, also called advanced or metastatic cancer, is not curable, so the aim of treatment is to relieve symptoms.

Find out more about treating breast cancer.

Living with breast cancer

Being diagnosed with breast cancer can affect daily life in many ways, depending on what stage it's at and the treatment you will have.

How people cope with the diagnosis and treatment varies from person to person.

There are several forms of support available, if you need it.

Forms of support may include:

- family and friends, who can be a powerful support system
- communicating with other people in the same situation
- finding out as much as possible about your condition
- not trying to do too much or overexerting yourself
- making time for yourself

Find out more about living with breast cancer.

Preventing breast cancer
As the causes of breast cancer are not fully understood, at the moment it's not possible to know if it can be prevented.

If you have an increased risk of developing the condition, some treatments are available to reduce your risk.

Studies have looked at the link between breast cancer and diet. Although there are no definite conclusions, there are benefits for women who:

- maintain a healthy weight
- exercise regularly
- have a low intake of saturated fat
- do not drink alcohol

It's been suggested that regular exercise can reduce your risk of breast cancer by almost as much as a third. Regular exercise and a healthy lifestyle can also improve the outlook for people affected by breast cancer. If you've been through the menopause, it's particularly important that you try to get to, and maintain, a healthy weight.
This is because being overweight or obese causes more oestrogen to be produced, which can increase the risk of breast cancer.
Macrobiotical Quisine and Joga
Macrobiotic diet

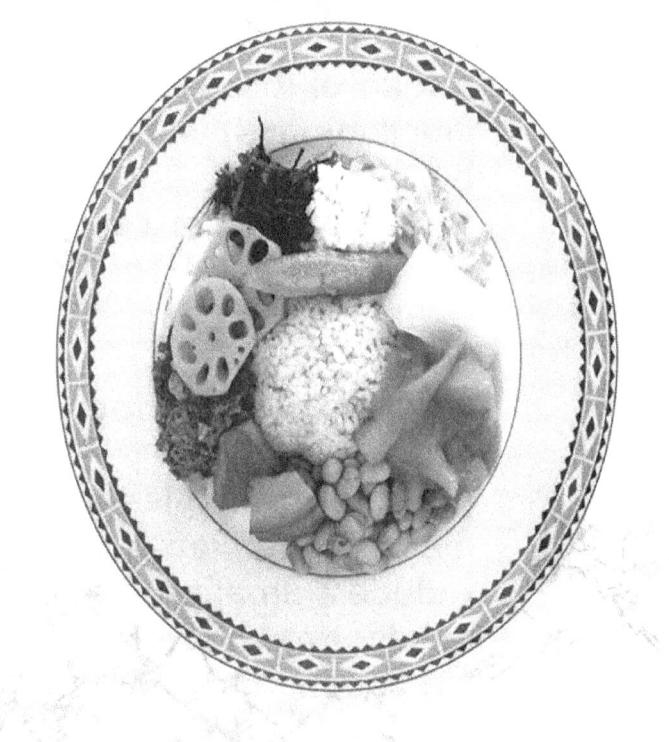

289

Subsequent proponents	George Ohsawa Michio Kushi William Dufty Edward Esko

A macrobiotic diet (or macrobiotics) is a fad diet based on ideas about types of food drawn from Zen Buddhism.[1][2] The diet tries to balance the supposed yin and yang elements of food and cookware.[1][3] Major principles of macrobiotic diets are to reduce animal products, eat locally grown foods that are in season, and consume meals in moderation.[2] There is no high-quality clinical evidence that a macrobiotic diet is helpful for people with cancer or other diseases, and it may be harmful.[4][2][5] Neither the American Cancer Society nor Cancer Research UK recommends adopting the diet. [6][5]

-
-
-
-
-
-
-

Conceptual basis

Macrobiotic diets are based on the concept of balancing yin and yang.[7]
The macrobiotic diet is associated with Zen Buddhism and is based on the idea of balancing yin and yang.[3] The diet proposes 10 plans which are followed to reach a supposedly ideal yin:yang ratio of 5:1.[7] The diet was popularized by George Ohsawa in the 1930s and subsequently elaborated on by his disciple Michio Kushi. [6] Medical historian Barbara Clow writes

that, in common with many other types of quackery, macrobiotics takes a view of illness and of therapy which conflicts with mainstream medicine.[8]

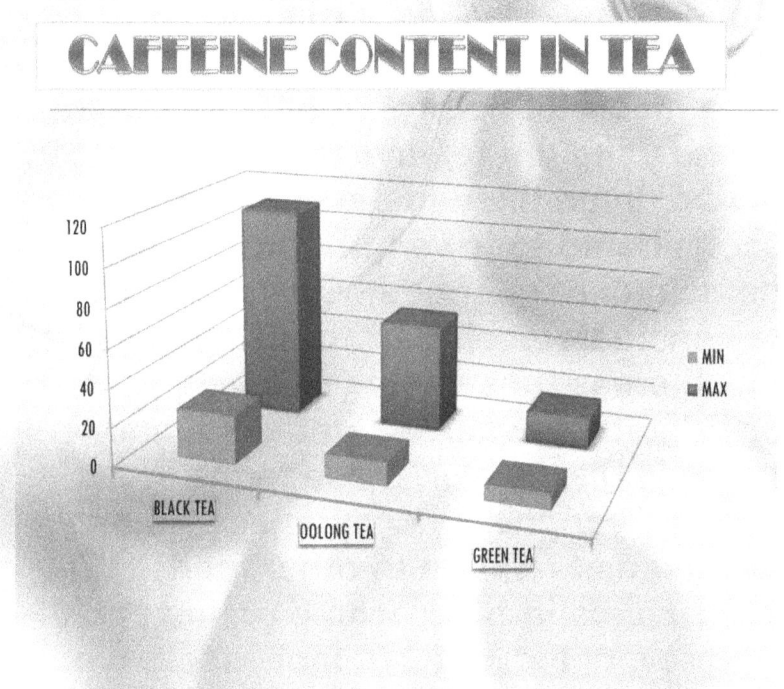

Macrobiotics emphasizes locally grown whole
grain cereals, pulses (legumes), vegetables, edible seaweed, fermented soy products, and fruit combined into meals according to the ancient Chinese principle of balance known as yin and yang.[9] Whole grains and whole-grain products such as brown rice and buckwheat pasta (soba), a variety of

cooked and raw vegetables, beans and bean products, mild
natural seasonings, fish, nuts and seeds, mild (non-stimulating) beverages such as bancha twig tea, and fruit are recommended.[10]
Some macrobiotic proponents stress that yin and yang are relative qualities that can only be determined in a comparison. All food is considered to have both properties, with one dominating. Foods with yang qualities are considered compact, dense, heavy, and hot, whereas those with yin qualities are considered expansive, light, cold, and diffuse.[11] However, these terms are relative; "yangness" or "yinness" is only discussed in relation to other foods.[12] Brown rice and other whole grains such as barley, millet, oats, quinoa, spelt, rye, and teff are considered by macrobiotics to be the foods in which yin and yang are closest to being in balance. Therefore, lists of macrobiotic foods that determine a food as yin or yang generally compare them to whole grains.[13]
Nightshade vegetables,
including tomatoes, peppers, potatoes, and eggplant; also, spinach, beets,

and avocados, are not recommended or are used sparingly in macrobiotic cooking, as they are considered extremely yin.[14] Some macrobiotic practitioners also discourage the use of nightshades because of the alkaloid solanine which is thought to affect calcium balance.[15] Some proponents of a macrobiotic diet believe that nightshade vegetables can
cause inflammation and osteoporosis.[16]
Practices
Food

Some basic macrobiotic ingredients
Some general guidelines for the Japanese-style macrobiotic diet are the following (it is also said that a macrobiotic diet varies greatly, depending on geographical and life circumstances):[17]
· Well-chewed whole cereal grains, especially brown rice: 40–60%
· Vegetables: 25–30%
· Beans and legumes: 5–10%

(-)-catechin (+)-epicatechin (-)-epigallocatechin

(-)-catechin-3-gallate (-)-epicatechin-3-gallate (-)-gallocatechin-3-gallate

(-)-epigallocatechin-3-gallate theaflavin

STRUCTURES OF TEA (CATECHINS)

theaflavin-3-gallate theaflavin-3,3'-digallate

- Miso soup: 5%
- Sea vegetables: 5%
- Traditionally or naturally processed foods: 5–10%

Fish and seafood, seeds and nuts, seed and nut butters, seasonings, sweeteners, fruits, and beverages may be enjoyed occasionally, two to three times per week. Other naturally-raised animal products may be included if needed during dietary transition or according to individual needs.

Kitchenware

Cooking utensils should be made from

certain materials such as wood or glass, while some materials including plastic, copper, and non-stick coatings are to be avoided.[1] Electric ovens should not be used.[1]

Japanese popularity and influence

The macrobiotic way of eating was developed and popularized by the Japanese. During the Edo period in Japan peasants had a diet based on staples of rice and soybeans. According to some macrobiotic advocates, a majority of the world population in the past ate a diet based primarily on grains, vegetables, and other plants. Because the macrobiotic diet was developed in Japan, Japanese foods that are thought to be beneficial for health are incorporated by most modern macrobiotic eaters.[18][19]

Cancer

The American Cancer Society recommends "low-fat, high-fiber diets that consist mainly of plant products"; however, they urge people with cancer not to rely on a dietary program as an exclusive or primary means of treatment.[6] Cancer Research UK states, "some people think living a macrobiotic lifestyle may help them to fight their cancer and lead to a cure. But there is no scientific evidence to prove this."[5]

Nutritionist Fredrick J. Stare has commented that "there is no scientific evidence that macrobiotic diets can be helpful for cancer or any other disease."[20]

Nutrition

The macrobiotic diet is a type of fad diet.[1][21] Most macrobiotic diets are not nutritionally sound.[7][22]

Fish provides vitamin B12 in a macrobiotic diet,[23] as bioavailable B12 analogues have not been established in any natural plant food, including sea vegetables, soya, fermented products, and algae.[24] Although plant-derived foods do not naturally contain B12, some are fortified during processing with added B12 and other nutrients.

[25] Vitamin A, as its precursor beta-carotene, is available from plants such as carrots and spinach.[26] Adequate protein is available from grains, nuts, seeds, beans, and bean products. Sources of Omega-3 fatty acids are discussed in the relevant article, and include soy products, walnuts, flax seeds, pumpkin seeds, hemp seeds, and fatty fish. Riboflavin along with most other B vitamins are abundant in whole

grains. Iron in the form of non-heme iron in beans, sea vegetables and leafy greens is sufficient for good health; detailed information is in the USDA database.[27]

Safety

Regulation

Macrobiotic practitioners are not regulated, and need not have any qualification or training in the United Kingdom.[5]

Complications

One of the earlier versions of the macrobiotic diet that involved eating only brown rice and water has been linked to severe nutritional deficiencies and even death. Strict macrobiotic diets that include no animal products may result in nutritional deficiencies unless they are carefully planned. The danger may be worse for people with cancer, who may have to contend with unwanted weight loss and often have increased nutritional and caloric requirements. Relying on this type of treatment alone and avoiding or delaying conventional medical care for cancer may have serious health consequences.[6]

Children

Children may also be particularly prone to nutritional deficiencies resulting from a macrobiotic diet.[6]

Pregnancy

Macrobiotic diets have not been tested in women who are pregnant or breast-feeding, and the most extreme versions may not include enough of certain nutrients for normal fetal growth.[6]

See also

· Ch'i
· Chinese food therapy
· List of diets
· List of unproven and disproven cancer treatments
· Sanpaku
· Shiatsu
· Traditional Chinese medicine

References

1.^ Jump up to:a b c d e Bijlefeld M, Zoumbaris SK (2014). Macrobiotics. Encyclopedia of Diet Fads: Understanding Science and Society (2nd ed.). ABC-CLIO. pp. 127–128. ISBN 978-1-61069-760-6.
2.^ Jump up to:a b c Lerman RH (7 December 2010). "The Macrobiotic Diet in Chronic Disease". Nutrition in Clinical Practice. 25 (6): 621–626. doi:10.1177/0884533610385704. PMID 21

139126.
3.^ Jump up to:a b Bender DA (2014). diet, macrobiotic. A Dictionary of Food and Nutrition. Oxford University Press. ISBN 9780191752391.
4.^ Hübner J, Marienfeld S, Abbenhardt C, Ulrich CM, Löser C (November 2012). "[How useful are diets against cancer?]". Deutsche Medizinische Wochenschrift (Review) (in German). 137 (47): 2417–22. doi:10.1055/s-0032-1327276. PMID 23152069.
5.^ Jump up to:a b c d "Macrobiotic diet". Cancer Research UK. Retrieved 8 July 2017.
6.^ Jump up to:a b c d e f Russell J; Rovere A, eds. (2009). "Macrobiotic Diet". American Cancer Society Complete Guide to Complementary and Alternative Cancer Therapies (2nd ed.). American Cancer Society. pp. 638–642. ISBN 9780944235713.
7.^ Jump up to:a b c Roth RA, Wehrle KL (2016). "Chapter 2: Planning a Healthy Diet". Nutrition & Diet Therapy (12th ed.). Cengage Learning. p. 43. ISBN 978-1-305-94582-1. The macrobiotic diet is a system of 10 diet plans, developed from Zen Buddhism

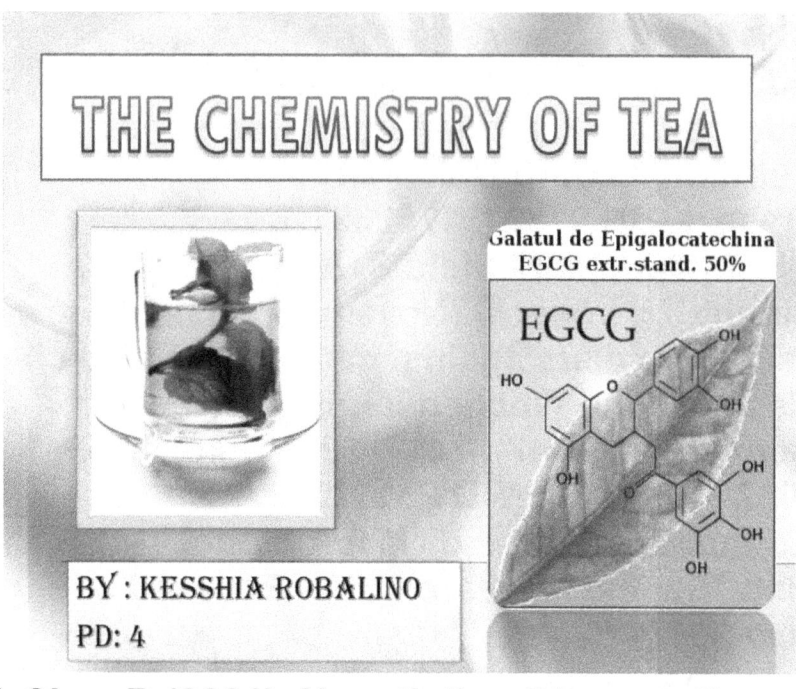

THE CHEMISTRY OF TEA

Galatul de Epigalocatechina
EGCG extr.stand. 50%

EGCG

BY : KESSHIA ROBALINO
PD: 4

8.^ Clow B (2001). Negotiating Disease: Power and Cancer Care, 1900-1950. McGill-Queen's University Press.
p. 63. ISBN 9780773522107.
Before we explore medical reactions to therapeutic innovations in this era, we must stop to consider the meaning of 'alternative medicine' in this context. Often scholars use the term to denote systems of healing that are philosophically as well as therapeutically distinct from regular medicine: homeopathy, reflexology, rolfing, macrobiotics, and spiritual healing, to name a few, embody interpretations of health, illness, and healing

that are not only different from, but also at odds with conventional medical opinion.

9. ^ William Dufty with Sakurazawa Nyoiti (1965) You Are All Sanpaku, University Books
10. ^ "Boiled Egg Diet". Retrieved 26 March 2016.
11. ^ Porter, pp. 22–25
12. ^ Porter, pp. 44–49
13. ^ Porter, pp. 71–78
14. ^ Kushi and Jack, p. 119.
15. ^ Stanchich L "All About Nightshades". New Life Journal: Carolina Edition, Apr/May 2003, vol. 4, no. 5, p. 17, 3 pp.
16. ^ Porter
17. ^ Kushi M; Blauer S; Esko W (2004). The Macrobiotic Way: The Complete Macrobiotic Lifestyle Book. Avery. ISBN 1-58333-180-8.
18. ^ Make Mine Macrobiotic | Lifestyle | Trends in Japan. Web Japan. Retrieved on 2012-04-27.
19. ^ Panel 11: Globalisation, Hybridity and Continuity in Traditional Japanese Health Practices. iastam.org
20. ^ Stare, Fredrick John; Whelan, Elizabeth M. (1998). Fad-Free Nutrition. Hunter House Inc. p. 127. ISBN 0-89793-237-4

21. ^ Hanning RM, Zlotkin SH (April 1985). "Unconventional eating practices and their health implications". Pediatr. Clin. North Am. (Review). 32 (2): 429–45. doi:10.1016/s0031-3955(16)34796-4. PMID 3887307.
22. ^ American Dietetic, Association; Dietitians Of, Canada (2003). "Position of the American Dietetic Association and Dietitians of Canada: Vegetarian diets". Journal of the American Dietetic Association. 103 (6): 748–765. doi:10.1053/jada.2003.50142. OCLC 1083 209. PMID 12778049. Vegetarian diets, like all diets, need to be planned appropriately to be nutritionally adequate.
23. ^ National Institutes of Health. "Dietary Supplement Fact Sheet: Vitamin B12". Retrieved 2008-05-27.

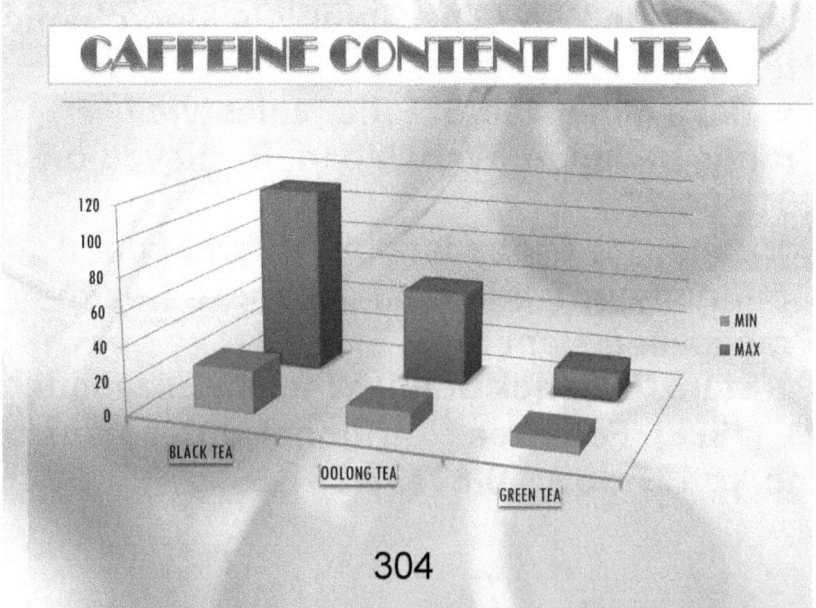

24. ^ USDA National Nutrient Database for Standard Reference, Release 20: Vitamin B-12 (μg) Content of Selected Foods per Common Measure, sorted by nutrient content.
25. ^ Reed Mangels. "Vitamin B12 in the Vegan Diet". Vegetarian Resource Group. Retrieved 2008-08-11.
26. ^ National Institutes of Health. "Dietary Supplement Fact Sheet: Vitamin A and Carotenoids (Table 2: Selected plant sources of vitamin A from beta-carotene)". Archived from the original on 2010-08-08. Retrieved 2008-05-28.
27. ^ USDA National Nutrient Database for Standard Reference, Release 20: Iron, Fe (mg) Content of Selected Foods per Common Measure, sorted by nutrient content.

Jump to nsa e varigca

h

t
i
o

n

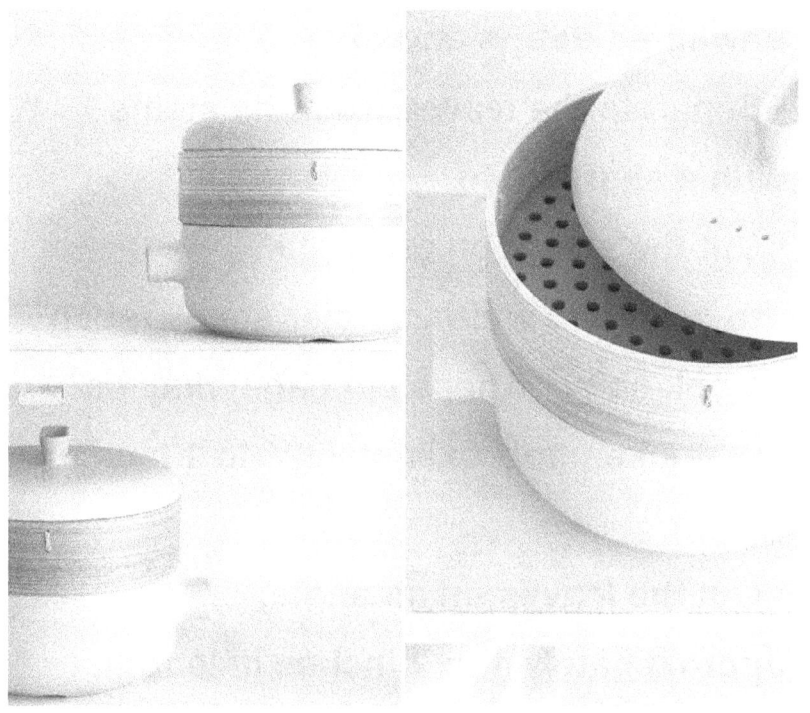

Macrobiotical recepies

unwanted debris and dirt.

• Separate the leaves from the stems with a sharp knife.

• Cut the stems on an angle.

to ¼ inch in width. Juicier stems (such as bok choy or napa cabbage) may be cut thicker, approximately ½ to 1 inch in length.

• Cut the leaves on an angle, approximately 1 to 2 inches in length.

• Place ¾ to 1 inch of water in the bottom of a pot and place the steamer basket over the pot.

• Cover and turn the flame to medium-high.

• When the pot is filled with steam, add the stems to the basket.

• Cover and steam for 20 seconds or

longer. The more fibrous the stem, the longer you will need to cook them, up to 1 minute in some cases.

• Add the leaves, cover and continue steaming for another 30 seconds or longer. Again, the texture of the greens varies according to the vegetable type, the growing season, and the environment.

• When done, the greens should still be crunchy, but tender enough to chew easily.

• Remove the greens from the basket and place in a serving dish. Cover with a sushi mat until serving.

• Optional: For an even lighter, more refreshing effect, add a squeeze of fresh lemon on your greens.

BLANCHED VEGETABLE SALAD

This light and colorful dish is a combination of root, round, and leafy green vegetables. The method of preparation and the combination of the different types of vegetables creates a dynamic energetic effect that helps to activate circulation from deep inside our bodies.

Preparation time: 10 to 15 minutes

Serves 2 to 3

Ingredients

• Choose a minimum of 2 different vegetables, from different categories, or use the combination listed below:

• 4 to 5 leafy greens, thinly sliced 1 inch wide by 2 inches in length

• 1 to 2 cups round vegetables, quartered and sliced thinly

• ½ cup root vegetables, cut into matchsticks ideally not thicker than ½ inch.

• A small pinch of sea salt

• Enough water to fill the pot halfway up

Cookware and Utensils

• A stainless-steel pot

• A spider or mesh vegetable skimmer (to remove vegetables from the water)

• Several plates

• Bamboo mats

Preparation

• Fill a pot halfway with water and bring the water to a boil over a medium flame.

• Add a pinch of sea salt.

• In an open pot, blanch one vegetable at a time, starting with the mildest in taste and lightest in color. When you add the vegetables, the water may stop boiling.

TSMD
e
o
i
o
a
g
s
r
g
p
r
e
l
c
a
e
a
h
c
y

t
F
I
S
n
u
i
r^{osle}epeat the process.
litn

•^{tsd} Repeat the entire process for all of the

n
r egetables.
e
T Allow the vegetables to cool, then
g
s
e
h
•en

312

g^Bently mix in a bowl.

•° Cover with a sushi mat until ready to serve.

• Optional: Sprinkle brown rice vinegar

or umeboshi vinegar on your blanched salad.

QUICK SAUTÉED VEGETABLES—RED ONION, BOK CHOY, CARROT
Preparation time: 10 to 15 minutes

Serves 4

Ingredients

• 1 medium onion, sliced in thin half-moons

• 1½ cups root vegetables, cut into thin matchsticks

• 4 to 6 leafy greens leaves, stems and leaves separated and cut ½ inch thick on the angle

• 1 to 2 teaspoons light sesame oil or 1 tablespoon extra virgin
olive oil

  teaspoon sea salt

• ¼ to ½ cup water

• Several drops shoyu

Note: Sautéed vegetables cook quickly. They should be bright, colorful, and crunchy.

Preparation

• Gently heat the oil in a saucepan, skillet, or other sautée pan.

• Tilt the pan so the oil spreads out evenly and lightly coats the bottom.

• Add the onions, turn up the flame, and begin to sautée.

• Add a little water, a pinch of sea salt, and continue to sautée for 2 minutes.

• Add the leafy green stems and more water if needed to keep the pan moist, continue to sautée.

• Add the leaves, followed by the root vegetables, and continue sautéeing.

• When the colors begin to deepen,

J u B m p O o B a c k N a v i g a t i o n

minutes, you are ready to season. Make sure you have a little juice in the bottom of the pan. If the pan is dry, add a little more water.

• Add a few drops of shoyu to the juice, then continue sautéeing to blend the seasoning.

• Remove the vegetables from the skillet, place in a serving dish, and cover with a sushi mat until ready to serve.

• Optional: Add a little spice, such as red pepper flakes or ginger juice. Chili pepper may be added after the onions at the beginning of cooking. A squeeze of fresh ginger juice may be added at the very end of cooking.

QUICK SAUTÉED LEAFY GREENS

This is a light preparation style where I begin by slightly steaming the greens, then adding oil and seasoning. The greens are juicy but still retain their crunchy texture.

Preparation time: 7 to 8 minutes

Serves 2 to 4

Ingredients

- ½ to 1 bunch leafy greens, washed and cut into larger pieces (approximately 2 to 3 inches in length and width). Baby greens may be kept whole.

teaspoon sea salt

- 1 tablespoon extra virgin olive oil or several drops of light sesame oil.
- If using olive oil, season only with sea salt.
- Season with 5 to 6 drops of shoyu if

using sesame oil.

Preparation

- Gently heat just enough water to cover the bottom of the pan.
- Add the stems, cover, and steam for 20 to 30 seconds.
- Add the leaves, cover, and steam for another 10 seconds.
- Drizzle a little oil over the top, then add a little sea salt and fold to blend the seasoning.
- Finish cooking the greens using a sautée method, approximately 20 to 30 more seconds. Place in a serving dish and

Turbo Charge Your Weight

Loss the Easy Way

Description

Let's be honest - dieting sucks and everyone hates it. Tasteless food, bird-like servings (that so often leave you hungry) and lackluster results that never last because, the truth is, most diets are not sustainable. The good news?

That's NOT what this book offers!

"Keto + Intermittent Fasting for Beginners" is a brief but comprehensive guide to the keto **lifestyle** and shows how incorporating the basic elements of intermittent fasting can make it even more powerful than it already is. This book will provide you with:

- The foundation of how the keto "diet" and intermittent fasting work and why they create such a powerful team.
- An understanding what ketosis is, why macros are important, and how to easily calculate and track yours.
- The guide to successfully lose weight, enjoy many other health benefits, and the solution to stop dieting forever.
- A 14-day meal plan (intermittent fasting is optional) – takes the guesswork out!
- 42 delicious and easy to follow recipes.
- Detailed shopping list.

Start losing weight and revitalizing your health today – you've got everything to gain!

legal or other professional advice or services. If professional assistance is required, the services of a competent professional person should be sought. Neither the Publisher nor the author shall be liable for damages arising herefrom. The fact that an individual, organization or website is referred to in this work as a citation and/or potential source of further information does not mean that the author or the publisher endorses the information the individual, organization or website may provide or recommendations they/it may make. Further, readers should be aware that Internet websites listed in this work may have changed or disappeared between when this work was written and when it is read.

Table of Contents

Introduction

Millions of people have hopped on the keto bandwagon in the last few years and it's easy to see why. Over the last several years the internet has been packed with images of before and after weight loss success stories, endorsements from A-list celebrities, and a compelling list of health benefits such as improved brain function and reduced cholesterol levels.

With keto you can forget about being limited to eating bland "diet" food, always being hungry, or seeing food as the enemy - like is so often experienced with other diets. Instead, keto will have you enjoying the rich flavours of real food and feeling satisfied at every meal.

Just like with anything new, there will be a time of adjustment as you develop the "chops" of eating keto. But you too can easily join the ranks of those who have successfully transitioned into the keto lifestyle.

You'll get there in no time….let's get started!

What is the Keto Diet?

Well, first of all it's not a diet. A diet is something you adopt temporarily, suffer through, and then abandon when you just "can't take it anymore". Am I right? Yeah, I can see more than a few heads nodding!

You may have heard it said before but, to repeat it - keto is not a diet, it's a lifestyle.

The reason we call it a lifestyle is because it's a way of eating that can be sustained, enjoyed, and incorporated into a permanent way of living. There is no starvation, no counting calories, and none of the "guilt" that comes with so many diets out there when all we want is to eat real satisfying and nourishing food!

With keto, you get to do that at every meal.

The basics of keto is that it's an eating plan based on whole and natural foods with an overall intake that is high in fat, moderate in protein and low in carbohydrates (think non starchy vegies).

You may notice that the USDA's Food Pyramid Guide is the exact opposite of that. It recommends severely limiting fats and heavily increasing carbohydrates to as much as 6 to 11 servings a day. And yet, since the Food Pyramid Guide was first released in 1980, studies show that rates of diabetes have skyrocketed from about 15% to 35% of all adults between the ages of 20 – 74. And, we all know that the obesity rates have increased dramatically as well.

Coincidence? I don't think so.

Let's just be clear that to maintain our health there are things called essential fatty acids and essential amino acids (protein). There is no such thing, however, as "essential carbohydrates".

Some studies have shown now that a diet high in carbohydrates can increase the risk conditions such as heart disease, obesity, depression, ADHD, mental health disorders, insulin resistance, pre-diabetes, metabolic syndrome, and eventually type II diabetes. Note; that is not an exhaustive list! Further, when

322

individuals experiencing some of these health issues adopt a low carb high fat diet, many of their conditions improve - some even disappear. While it goes against the "education" we've been subjected to now for decades, it's key to understand that most naturally occurring fats are good for us and are not the evil culprit of obesity and disease in the way that we have been brainwashed into believing.

Weight Loss – Just the Tip of the Ice Burg

It may surprise you to know that the "Keto Diet" is not some latest and greatest new fad diet that some weight loss guru has just invented. It's actually been around for a long time. And, it was not developed with weight loss in mind. The ketogenic diet was originally developed in the 1920s as a strictly therapeutic protocol for children suffering from epilepsy. It was very successful but unfortunately the medical community's love affair with pharmaceutical drugs took over and the ketogenic diet fell back into the shadows.

In more recent years, the ketogenic diet has been the subject of many scientific studies and has been put back into the spotlight for the positive results showing in many areas like:

*Weight Loss

*Increased mental clarity

*Improved memory

*Therapeutic treatments for autism and dementia

*Alzheimer's prevention

*Decreasing blood pressure

*Improved cholesterol levels

*Sustained increase in energy and vitality

*Improved complexion

*Improved sleep

*Longevity

*Treatment for depression

*Treatment for diabetes

*Stabilizing hormones - improving fertility, PCOS symptoms

*Preventing/reversing pre-diabetes and type II diabetes

*Anti-Inflammatory effects – reducing joint pain, arthritis, psoriasis

Compelling list, right?

For many people, their primary reason for embarking on the keto lifestyle is for weight loss. But, as you can see, the benefits are more far-reaching than just that one thing. Keto is a way of eating and a lifestyle that the whole family can embark on and benefit from together.

What Is Ketosis & Why Do I Want It?

Ok, here's the sciencey stuff.

Now, it's certainly not necessary at all to have a PhD in all things keto science in order to succeed with it. But I feel it really helps in creating the new habits of keto when we understand even just a tiny bit of what's actually happening behind the scenes.

Understanding the basic biology of the "what and why" of ketosis goes a long way when we find ourselves staring down a bag of Doritos. Knowing some of the science will help you win that face-off every time!

But, don't worry. I won't go into nutty detail that will make you feel like you're back in science class! And, there won't be a test at the end – promise...

So, the premise is very counter-intuitive. Eat fat to lose fat? What? But yes, that is exactly how it works. And here is just a little of the wonderful sciencey stuff that will show you why.

By eating the keto way, it changes the way our body converts food into energy. When we eat carbohydrates, our body breaks down the carbs (think bread, pasta, potatoes) into glucose for energy. Our system will choose this energy source as it's first choice because it's the most easily accessible. But our system can only take so much glucose floating around. Once all our immediate energy needs are met, any excess glucose is stored as fat. Now, all that energy is locked up in our fat stores (and likely forming that muffin top we all love so much).

In not too long, we eat again, and supply our body with a fresh dose of carbs. Our system will once again use the free-flowing glucose for immediate energy first, the excess will be stored as fat. And, oh... hang on a second.

Here comes another high carb meal! And on and on we go....

With a high carbohydrate diet it can be very difficult to use up those fat stores for energy because our systems will always use the free-flowing glucose first. When we don't have free-flowing glucose in our system something wonderful happens. In the absence of free glucose in the system, our bodies are forced to find energy elsewhere. So, it begins to break down and convert fat into something called ketones and uses that for energy.

This is the metabolic process called ketosis.

When we stay in this state of ketosis, our bodies use dietary fat, protein, and stored fat as a primary source of fuel. This is bad news for the muffin top and great news for you!

Intermittent Fasting – It's Not as Weird as You Think

Intermittent fasting has become rather popular recently. But, it's not new – it's even older than the ketogenic diet. Fasting has been included as part of everyday life for eons across all cultures and religions. Historically, many associations with fasting have been spiritual in nature but many have also incorporated the health-giving properties that ancient people and cultures seemed to have understood instinctively.

Actually, fasting is not new for any of us. We all fast. From the time we stop eating at night to the time we eat breakfast the next day we are fasting. The word "breakfast" says it all – with our first meal in the morning we are literally breaking our fast.

The only difference with intermittent fasting is that it's simply done with more intention. Rather than an 8 hour-ish window of "accidental" fasting while we sleep, we purposely increase that to a 12, 16, 18 hour fast, or more.

There are several different ways in which people practice intermittent fasting. It can be as simple as delaying the first meal of the day until lunch every day or as involved as cycling different fasting periods in differing lengths of time throughout the month, some as long as 24-72 hours or more.

Please note: As the purpose of this book is to serve the keto and intermittent fasting beginner, we will be focusing only on the simple applications of intermittent fasting. We will not address the more advanced strategies of intermittent fasting.

Most of us have probably been raised with the adage that "breakfast is the most important meal of the day". I know I was. But... that's actually not true. Delaying your first meal until later in the day is a great way to incorporate intermittent fasting into your daily routine.

You might already be doing this without meaning to. I know a lot of people who skip breakfast because they don't have time in their hectic morning or even because eating first thing in the morning doesn't agree with them. If that's you, you don't have to change a thing! If it's not you, don't worry. It's much easier than you may think.

Even our modern science backs up the ancient's belief in and practice of fasting. Studies show that fasting can (among other things):

*Ward off chronic disease

*Lower insulin levels

*Improve memory and brain function

*Improve cholesterol counts

*Reduce inflammation

*Boost our metabolism

*Increase energy levels

Even more, intermittent fasting is a powerful way to lose weight and keep it off.

While 12, 16 or 18 hours may sound like a long time to go without eating, don't worry. It's important to note that your body will still get all the food and nutrition it needs but just during a shorter period of time.

Keto + Intermittent Fasting = The Dynamic Duo

These two work wonders together!

Intermittent fasting is a great support to keto as it helps anyone get into the state of ketosis faster. And, it helps us to remain in a state of ketosis as well. That is always a great thing because ketosis = fat burning magic!

Keep in mind that intermittent fasting is NOT necessary to reach ketosis or to have success and great results with the keto lifestyle. There are even some people who can't fast for health reasons. This is completely fine. Incorporating intermittent fasting with keto is an option, not a requirement.

But, because it's such a very powerful combination for most people, I wanted to be sure that I included it in this book so that you'd know how to incorporate intermittent fasting with your keto plan.

How to Include Intermittent Fasting with Keto

There are different versions and a variety of different ways to "do" intermittent fasting. As this is a beginner's guide, we will stick to the more straight- forward methods.

1) **16/8 Method:** This is typically the "skip breakfast" method giving you a 16 hour window to fast and an 8 hour window to eat. Doing this method is as simple as not eating anything after dinner, skipping breakfast the next morning, and having your first meal at lunch. Effectively, you eat 2 meals a day.

Example: Stop eating by 8 pm on Monday and have your next meal at 12 noon on Tuesday.

(Note: it is usually recommended that women adjust this fast to a 14/10 or 15/9 as women seem to do better with slightly shorter fasts)

2) **5:2 Method:** This method involves eating normally 5 days a week and doing a low calorie "fast" 2 days a week. The 24 hour fasting days for women would include eating 500 calories and for men 600. (2 small meals a day of 250 for women and 300 for men).

Naturally, when doing this method, you should space the fasting days evenly.

Example: Low calorie "fast" on Monday and Thursday, eat normally on all other days.

3) **Eat-Stop-Eat Method:** This method involves fasting for a full 24 hours once or twice a week and was made popular by fitness expert Brad Pilon. Fasting from one dinner one day to dinner the next day = 24 hours. You can fast from any meal – breakfast to breakfast; lunch to lunch; dinner to dinner. Your choice.

During the fasting period you can drink water, coffee, tea or other non-caloric beverages
but no solid food. Spread the fasting days evenly through the week 3 or
4 days apart.

Example: Fast on Monday and Thursday, eat normally on all other days.

- If you're using intermittent fasting as part of your weight loss plan, it's important to eat normally at your next meal. Don't go crazy and eat enough for 3 people!
- During any fasting period make sure to maintain adequate water intake.
- Adding another element to keto can be intimidating for many, especially for those who are new to keto. If that's you, not to
worry! One of the best ways to get all the benefits of keto and intermittent fasting AND remove all the overwhelm is to have someone else do all the work in figuring it out for you. Finding a "done-for-you program" to use and follow is a perfect solution

Keto Coffee

Many will know this by the name "bulletproof coffee".

That term is actually a trademarked brand so I use the term keto coffee to describe as it's very popular among the keto community.

Keto-style coffee is coffee with MCT oil and butter. Some people will also add a little heavy whipping cream. It will give you the pep of caffeine, the brain- boosting benefits of the MCT oil and the energy sustaining effects of the butter.

If putting butter in your coffee sounds weird to you. I get it. It did to me too the first time I heard about it and I avoided it for quite a while. But, it's nice! I bet you'll be pleasantly surprised.

There isn't really a "right" way to make keto coffee. You can do it to taste. Some people find their digestive systems respond better to a gradual introduction to MCT oil so start easy with just ½ teaspoon per cup.

Anytime is a great time for a keto coffee. Just be mindful that many people find caffeine can disrupt their sleep if taken too far into the afternoon.

Plan to Win – Success Leaves Clues

"If you fail to plan you are planning to fail."

Benjamin Franklin

"Success leaves

clues." Jim Rohn

Take a page out of the book of both highly esteemed and accomplished gentlemen.

To succeed with keto**, let's**

plan… **Step 1: Keto Kitchen**

Cleanse

Grab a shopping bag and head to your cupboards, fridge, and freezer. Anything non keto goes into the bag. Things like, croutons, ketchup, bread, pasta, BBQ sauce, cookies, crackers, cereal, syrup, jelly, candy, juice, salad dressing….etc. Read the labels of all these items and you may be surprised to find how many things are hiding enormous amounts of sugar. Take the bag of loot and drop off the non-perishables at your local food bank, gift things from your fridge and freezer to family, friends and co-workers. Or, you can do them a favour too and just toss them and leave them curbside on garbage day.

If it's not in your house, you can't eat it. Simple.

Now, I can hear many of you saying "But, my spouse/kids/roommate live here too. They aren't doing keto. I can't throw away all their favourite food!" If that's you, make sure you clearly explain that you're doing keto, what that

329

means in terms of what you do and do not eat, and most importantly WHY you're doing it and WHY it means a lot to you. By doing this you are allowing them to more effectively support you. Figure out a compromise together. Such as, they bring less of "that" kind of food into the house. The stuff that is there maybe can be moved to a different area of the house or kitchen. When I got to do this, I negotiated for the foods I had the most challenge with resisting to be kept in a very high cupboard above the fridge. This was effective for me because I'm very short. The effort and focus I'd have to put into getting into that cupboard allowed me the time to "snap out of it" and make a different choice. (drag a chair across the kitchen, climb up, stand on my tip toes, strain to reach the cupboard…. you get the picture!)

By making your home as keto friendly as possible you're planning to succeed!

Step 2: Plan Your Meals

To avoid accidental or emergency non-keto meals, plan your menu for the week. This way you won't succumb to something like the lure of fast food when you realize at 7 pm on a Tuesday night that the fridge is empty and you have no idea what to do for dinner.

Many people find they like to do this on a Saturday or Sunday. Plan your menu for the following Monday to Sunday. Choose each meal for each day, check your macros, write it down, collect the recipes, make a shopping list, head to the store, stock the fridge. Now, you've taken all the guesswork out of it. You've already made all your meal decisions so the rest of the week it's easy peasy!

By planning your meals for the week ahead of time you're planning to succeed!

Step 3: Attitude and Mind Set

Choose to be excited about the changes you've decided to make by going keto. We can't control many things in this world but the one thing we can control is our attitude. You will have challenging moments as you make the transition to keto but decide now that you will approach each challenge with a positive and empowered mind set.

Make sure that you're really connected with your WHY of going keto and all the benefits you want to enjoy. Remember what it was that you were unhappy with that led you to make the decision for keto in the first place. Was it to feel more confident with your appearance? To get off the path to diabetes your Dr. told you that you were headed towards.? To have more energy so you could play with your kids for more than 10 minutes at a time? To be able to bend down to tie your shoes and breathe at the same time? You can make it just as difficult or as easy as you wish. Choose easy! By keeping your attitude in check, you're planning to succeed!

Step 4: Support System

Tell those around you what you are doing! Don't keep keto a secret. That's just silly. Let those closest to you in on your lifestyle change. Tell them what kinds of food you will and will not be eating on keto. And…tell them WHY you are making this lifestyle change – ask them for their support.

If people understand how meaningful this is to you, they will me much more able to step up and support you. When people don't understand your "why" that's when they're more likely going to try to talk you into eating all the stuff you used to eat. "Oh, come on…just one bite won't hurt you!" Help them to help you. Let them in on it.

Get around like-minded people! Even if you're the only person in your house doing keto it doesn't mean you have to do it alone. With social media it's super easy to get into a community of people who are on the same journey as you are. Communities and group support are so powerful when it comes to inspiration, accountability, support and social connection.

I run a private group on Facebook that delivers just that. People share their stories, their keto achievements and challenges, tips and tricks, and I get in there too on a regular basis and do open keto Q&A's.

Consider this your official invitation to join us there – for FREE!

Come hang out with me!

By providing yourself a support system you are planning to succeed!

Tracking Your Macros

It's important to note the exact ratios will depend on each person's activity level, your actual weight and how your body responds to this eating plan. The amount of protein and fat consumed can vary a little but most people enjoy the best and most consistent results by keeping the amount of carbohydrate limited to about 20 - 30 grams a day.

(20 gms = ideal; 30 gms = max)

Carbs – carbs should be consumed for micronutrient delivery (ie: vitamins/minerals) and enjoyment. A good target is to limit your daily carb intake to 20 grams. This is universal and isn't affected by gender, height or weight.

Protein – daily intake of protein depends upon lean body mass so will vary from person to person and is affected by gender, height, weight and activity level.

Figuring out your lean body mass will help you understand how to target your protein intake. For the average person, with an average activity level, that will be about .7g to .8g of protein per lb of lean body mass. *(how to calculate your lean body mass is on the next page)*

Fat – daily fat intake has a relationship with the amount of protein you eat and is consumed and adjusted according to hunger and energy needs. It's pretty simple - eat fat to satiety (until your hunger is satisfied).

Often, this will work out on the low side to be around a 1:1 ratio and on the high side around a 2:1 ratio of fat to protein.

When it comes to fat intake, you get to listen to your body. If you are fully satisfied having eaten to a 1:1 ratio of fat/protein...great! If you're still really hungry then go ahead and eat more fat.

We are not wanting to have you stay in a legitimately hungry state – that is not required (or advised… a cookie binge won't be far behind!).

Be satisfied!

Here is an example of the calculations completed for a person who determined they had a lean

body mass of 100 lbs:

- Carb Calculation: 20g a day
- Protein Calculation:

Lean body mass is 100 lbs x .7g (or .8g)

= 70g to 80g of protein a day.

- Fat Calculation:

Protein intake is 70g to 80g a day

= 70g to 80g of fat a day for a 1:1 ratio

= 140g to 160g of fat a day for a 2:1 ratio

This person now has their daily targets for all 3 macronutrients:

Carbs: 20 grams

Protein: 70 – 80 grams

Fat: 1:1 ratio: 70 – 80 grams

2:1 ratio: 140 – 160 grams

Please keep in mind this is a general average. For instance, people who are very active and athletic may likely need to eat closer to 1g of protein per lb of lean body mass. Others who are very insulin sensitive may find they do better eating .6g of protein per lb of lean body mass. For the purposes of this conversation, we're keeping it simple by using the general average of . 7g

to .8g per lb.

How To Calculate Your Lean Body Mass

Let's clarify how lean body mass is defined. Basically, it is everything minus body fat. So, the skeleton, ligaments, organs, blood vessels, cartilage etc. … this is what makes up our lean body mass.

There are a bunch of different ways to calculate lean body mass. Some people use fat calipers, but they can be difficult to use properly and are quite inaccurate if you have a lot of excess fat. For the adventurous, there are high-tech methods such as hydrostatic weighting or a dexa scan (measures bone density and body composition).

But, the easiest way to calculate your personal approximate lean body mass is to use an online US Navy calculator. Just Google "us navy calculator" and punch in your basic info. This won't be an exact calculation, but it will be moderately accurate and can be done quickly and easily. Here is one such calculator:

http://fitness.bizcalcs.com/Calculator.asp?Calc=Body-Fat-Navy

Don't Get Along With Math?

For those of you who have a relationship with math that falls under "it's complicated" status, don't despair! Figuring out your daily targets for all 3 macros is happily not something you have to do all the time! Once you figure out what those macro targets are, all that is needed from there is to track them each day.

Keep in mind that NOT tracking your macros is a strategy destined for failure. So please… don't ignore this part of things.

Tracking carbs "ish" is not a strategy!

The only way to get away with not tracking your macros, that I can personally recommend, is to take advantage of this proven keto program.

To your keto success!!

General Keto Food Staples

While not an exhaustive list, here are many of the basic foods and ingredients that will support you in your new keto lifestyle.

Vegetables

Asparagus

Broccoli

Cauliflower

Lettuce

Kale

Artichoke

Celery

Zucchini

Yellow Squash

Bell Peppers

Keto + Intermittent Fasting For Beginners: to fuperfast Cancer even in progressed stages

Your Local Reverend

Introduction I now as Asoka would like to express myself to general welbeing in the Czech Republic and I came up with the following. I would introduce wages 4xtimes 15 000 crowns a month with a central banking, working on the bases of Irish and American paypal. A preprogramed website incorporated into main platform from which you can each week gain your wage social income for bettering general welbeing. the whole system of social income should afterwards became fully digital on a sms and one card. Radichemotherapy is a treatment of cancer which makes you feel sick and people from this treatment die either during treatment or within two months after treatment. Sickness, nausea, loose stools during radiochemotherapy or post-treatment time can be affected by supplementary medication (Haliperdidol, etc..) The problem of this treatment is that it is not effective, but radiochemotherapy has spread within the last 20 years all over the Czech Republic and has been widely professed on dosens of people. Several of my friends died of chemotherapy and my Aunt Leeba or Ishka had intestinal cancer due to complaints on abdomenal and itestinal pains. Why they were not adviced by doctor to use for example Glivnol, or other ointments nobody understands. The treatment of cancer over the last 15 years in the Czech Republic has reachd the dimensions of creating facilities not dissimilar to Lagres where all women supposedly aflected by this desease are tested and gived doesens of newly introduced or still developing pills. Why the czech Republic has never introduced the Biomedical pills developed in Thaiwan or macrobiotical quisine with additional welfare for this treatment (200 000 dollars) has no conclusion, except that they profess Chemotherapy on people to extort moneyy from the afflicted and ultimately kill out all your family and pillage the House and the bank accounts. Cancer is also used as a blackmail for money. Mari who inherited fields and 50 000 000 was given radiochemotherapy and died within two months. The problem is also in sexual hedony as people through the widespread of computers and telefones use these gadgets for inner mantal masturbation and doctors are thus sexually ruptured from extorig and, pillage and murder. All these aligations are here by me stated and given as I now profer you all these prooves for this 'medical' method to be eradicated and and I also ask the Epam by Boris Jarkovsky and Tibetian Medicine supposedly desregarded my Prsident Milosh Zeman be sent and given to medical and biomedical laboratories for carrying on in, and enlivening the trade from the ast and the Himalayas and all these intments and creames be further developed into fully-fledgen medicaments. These progneses are my prognoses for the 21st Century, carryed out in the homage of Srtre and Astrid Lindgren and other people whe devoted their lives, or layed their lives for the benefit of the Society. Also now, in terms of Papeu new Guinea, that by Rawra investigated for wa widespread occurance of unbleamised pristine granite rocks, and beds should according to Rawra lead into building on these secluded pristine places Toxic waste and irridium and pottasium storidges – is now by me desregarded. As I believe that Paopua new Guinea should be in fact, if anything, be carred outinto a fledgen cities and skysrapers witha wider population densety carryed out predominantly by Austarian power and the power of of its Judislature. As here I now therefore reprimand Rawra for blemishing the work, memory and reprimand given by Sir. David Ettenborough and his wede proofs for his late dvindeling of the the ocean strip and habitat. Benjamin (Allan) Schmidt (Asoka) Breast tumor fire basically spazms which can be cause by spastic sleep from medication or overmedication, bad glucose contained in anticonception, or spazmic sleep caused from anticonception, brain uncers are thus caused from deprived brain and dehidration. Vitamin A - sight Vitamin B - skin and healing Vitamin C - healing and revitalising and hidrating (old for cancer and true) All these vitamins are contained in Bergamot. By creating separate vitamines in a Mof and chanelling them on protons we can create a boxfor bombarding which should - relax and releave deranged metabolism and heal tumors, ulcers or maligne spots. It is interesting to porn out that wecould also create a hand machine that works on the bases of a Mof precipitator to locally distil calcifications and spazmas. Ia nowve closetotheinvesflgaflonof cancer-InowbeHevethatCancerisa veneraldeseaseprocuredduring intercoursefrorSperr.ItisanAf can deseaseprefarabelyaRacldngcocassions duetoi uni proble s. Cancer can also erase in womans shlem, but not so o£en like in men's sperm can result into far reaching health rammifications. Healing proteins and *enzymes from Ku a and bancha treated int a(cine can obliterate the ask and create a lifelo immunity cancer bacteria African j?jvater Vipassanii Meditation Para Nirvana Nirvana i Thought (samatha) Thoughts Conceptual Thinking Living God 1,a cm hair Half Lotus Posture Generator of Money Sv6sidiary Bank-link monitor with payyal adder, batcain adder and credit card Slot far a credit*

.